THE CANNABIS SOLUTION

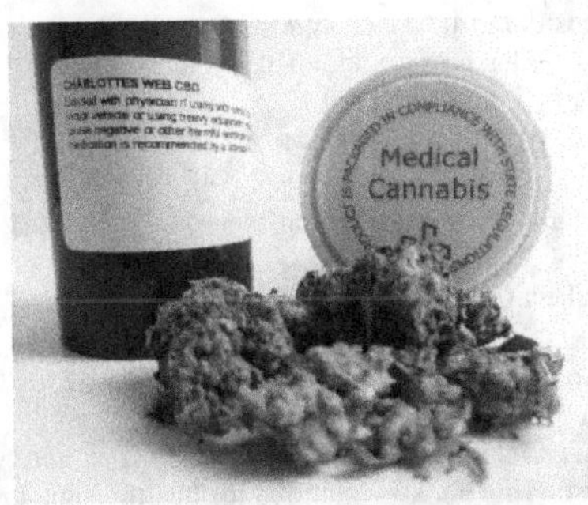

WHAT THEY DON'T WANT YOU TO KNOW ABOUT

Arkansas Edition

Dr. Tammy Post

For information about permissions to reproduce selections from this book or to purchase copies for educational, business or sales promotional use, contact:

BETTER LIVING RX
www.BETTERLIVINGRX.com
Email: info@betterlivingrx.com

Lily Grace Publishing Ltd.

Published by Lily Grace Books, a Division of Parks-Haas House Inc., New York

DEDICATION

To those who have been fighting the good fight against the "War on Weed" and sought to undo the fear surrounding one of them most diverse and healing plants God has ever given to us. To those who know that "reefer madness" was just a political ploy to keep us terrified of the gifts of the Ganga and in the dark about the possibilities for a better quality of life.

ACKNOWLEDGMENTS

To the universe for knowing what we need before we can or will acknowledge that we need it!

CONTENTS

Foreword By Wendy Love Edge

I was introduced to Dr. Tammy on social media. She was giving free live feed seminars about a variety of health topics including stem cells, hormones and medicinal cannabis. I was intrigued that a Doctor would take the time to do this. This is important, because social media in 2017 is a primary tool that the general public uses to obtain information. And here was a trained Medical Doctor willing to take the time to share their expertise and information! I reached out to her, after reviewing her credentials. I found she was not only a well-trained Family Medicine Doctor who specializes in functional and wellness medicine, bio-identical hormone therapy, anti-aging, metabolic genetic testing and therapeutic intervention, alternative medical therapy, nutrition and exercise physiology, but she is also an author, speaker, integrative medicine consultant and wellness expert!

Additionally, to my delight, I realized that she was another physician who had opted out of the giant money and greed mill of the pharmaceutical and the insurance industries. The industries that tied Doctors hands from offering patients anything but pills, tests, and surgery.

I understood this twisted situation first hand. In 2011, after being treated for many years for several autoimmune diseases by pharmaceutical products, I became gravely ill with an autoimmune disease called dermatomyositis. I became "bulldozed" by the healthcare system and told that I would die from the disease or the drugs they had to give me to treat it. I believed them. Because of this fact, I did everything they told me. I soon found myself in a power wheelchair, unable to care for myself and on 16 pharmaceutical drugs. The treatment got me out of the acute phase, but repeatedly I was told I couldn't come off of the drugs that I was on, despite wanting to improve my life and my functional abilities. I improved enough to walk on arm crutches, but I was just surviving. I couldn't drive, I was confused and had major memory and emotional issues, and worst of all, I had no hope. I was also in and out of the hospital once a month due to an ailing immune system. This "treatment" was ineffectual because it did not equal well care, or a positive quality of life. It created more dis-ease and side effects rendering me feeling unwell most of the time, and just surviving. Survival does not equal quality living. It is simply surviving.

In 2013, I went through a personal transformation. I changed my mind, deciding that I could improve my health. I then made the decision without my doctor's knowledge, to start weaning off of as many of the pharmaceutical drugs that I had been taking. I didn't know I was addicted to opiates, benzodiazepines, and many other drugs until I started to come off of them. I soon entered the withdrawal process. In full withdrawal, sweating, shaking and unable to control the anxiety, depression and pain, I was desperate to keep going and find an alternative. A friend suggested that I try medicinal cannabis. I responded, "You want me to get high? How is that productive to this process? I'm trying to see what I have left and if I can get out of survival mode and into a life." She replied calmly, "Let's look up the medicinal properties. I think it will help you." And so we did. I am a woman of science. I had received my Bachelor of Science in Occupational Therapy, graduating magna cum laude from Boston University in 1987. I needed proof. Though the studies are limited in the U.S. due to many factors of greed, ignorance and the tyranny of pharmaceutical companies, the government and the FDA, there were articles for me to review. I was also reaching a desperation point with the withdrawal symptoms. Maybe I just needed my own anecdotal evidence. If I improved, even if it was the placebo effect, it would be a welcomed change. Finally, I agreed to smoke some cannabis with my friend, who admittedly had been an avid recreational and medicinal user most of her life. The pain and withdrawal symptoms disappeared almost entirely with the first few puffs. Hope began to well up inside me in that instant. I knew that cannabis was my medicine.

What followed, was me figuring out that even in a legal state, the system was difficult to navigate and mainstream doctors weren't permitted to write recommendations if they took any federal funding. For instance, if they accepted Medicare (and most of them do) they couldn't write the recommendation.

Since I had already changed my mind and was determined to improve my life and health, I pushed through and found avenues to become legal. The cannabis was healing my body and mind. I had withdrawn successfully from 7 pharmaceutical drugs in 30 days using cannabis and was continuing that process. It opened my mind and creativity. I saw possibilities where before I saw walls and barriers. I had more energy and started improving my lifestyle with proper nutrition, meditation and exercise. I saw a chiropractor and other complementary health professionals. I also realized quickly that everything I wanted to do for true health, I had to pay for out of my pocket. I could easily have gone to the pharmacy at any time and obtained the pills prescribed for next to nothing out of my pocket. But the cannabis doctor, the cannabis medicine, the complementary providers, even healthy food was barely available to me on my budget. It was all a classist system, accessible only to those with the money. I was not a conspiracy theorist, but it seemed to me that the pharmaceutical companies, the insurance industry and the government were not interested in true health. It seemed that they had every citizen who hadn't woken up to this fact, under their control. Many blindly staring at their cell phones, eating processed food, ingesting pills daily and never getting out from under their piles of bills for health care that was ineffectual.

I decided to start a nonprofit organization, to help everyone achieve health and wellness by providing access and education. I called it Bulldozer Health Inc., and we obtained 501c3 status in 2014. It continues to grow today out of the efforts of many passionate people. As for my own health, I still have my struggles and so-called diseases. I try very hard not to live into them and to do everything in my power to achieve a maximal level of wellness. I can't erase the 49 years of pharmaceutical drugs, and then pharmaceutical overload, and unhealthy lifestyle that is in my past. I can only continue to do everything in my power to improve my health and well being, and inspire others to do the same. Cannabis is still my medicine today, and without it, I know that my quality of life would plummet. The field of regenerative medicine, or stem cells also inspires me. I am greatly encouraged that is a treatment also that Dr. Tammy is pursuing.

So, when I saw Dr. Tammy on social media, I knew we had to have her as a part of our organizations health network. Through our health network we can help individuals access providers, by paying for their treatment as our fundraising and donations allow. Network providers also provide education on our larger format. The general population needs access to complementary health methods, but also innovative treatments from their physician based in science. That is what Dr. Tammy offers! And so naturally, she is offering evaluation and recommendations to patients who will benefit from medicinal cannabis through her clinics.

In this book, you will read success stories of patients like me, who improved their health via the natural method of ingesting cannabis medicine in its many forms. Some of the patients, or their loved ones, were in life threatening situations. May they inspire you to go forward and speak the truth of the healing properties of medicinal Cannabis. When you do this, like Dr. Tammy and myself, you are working to break the stigma created by greed and untruths that is still prevalent in the U.S. and other countries today. Much gratitude to Dr. Tammy, for stepping forward and extending the reach and voice of those who have found improved health with cannabis medicine.
In Peace and Love,
Wendy Love Edge
Founder, Bulldozer Health Inc. www.bulldozerhealth.org
 Take back your health America!

Introduction

Who Are You?

If you are reading this you are probably either curious, frustrated with some illness that has had no adequate relief with traditional treatments, or the friend or family member of someone who is seeking non-traditional treatment and they have handed you this book in an attempt to alleviate your fears or concerns about their interest or usage of medical cannabis. Who ever you are we hope to allay your fears, deliver the facts and empower you through education and understanding of options available. Knowledge is power!

Who am I?

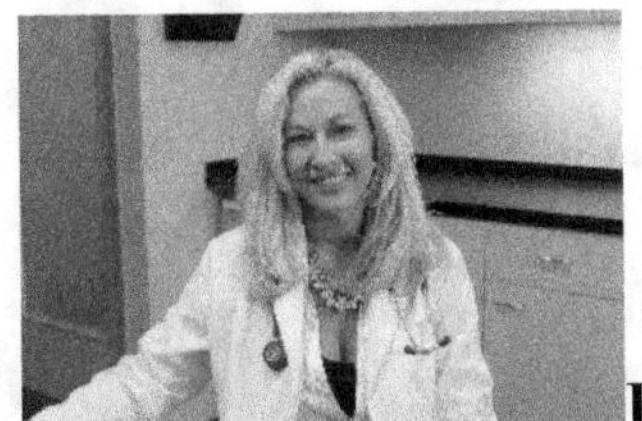

Dr. Tammy Post

How does a doctor who has always viewed marijuana as a terrible drug that consumes the youth bridges a gateway into the underworld of destructive behaviors of insidious narcotics usage, heroin, meth, acid or alcoholism that leaves its victims hopelessly strung out addicted dregs on society get into the world of medical cannabis you may ask? I started out this journey through a very naive and idealistic view of the medical world. My first thoughts of becoming a doctor were as a little girl. Doctoring my stuffed animals, performing surgery on them, bandaging their boo-boos and kissing them on the foreheads when they were sick. Holes daunted their mouths for thermometers and I learned to use a needle and thread very early to stich them. I had an obsession with tape and bandages so often you could see little of their little bear or doggie faces peering out from mummy like wraps. My mother planted these seeds much earlier by investing in medical encyclopedias for my older brothers (eight and sixteen years older in fact) that they might purse the prestigious profession that secure her financial retirement privileges. My brothers were a bit of a disappointment in that regard but somehow the seed took in fertile soil with me. My first exposure to Marijuana was my older brother who sought distraction from the world as a teenager and thanks to "reefer madness" my parents were sufficiently terrified that he would become at best a "pot-head" and at worst a drug addicted derelict, hopelessly lost and more of a disappointment than just missing the boat to becoming a physician. As the years passed I was rarely ever exposed to any sort of peer pressure of drugs as I was way to fearful to ever disappoint my parents. No, I would be the good girl and become their every expectation so I used judgment and justification against those that imbibed in any sort of alcohol or drugs. I didn't even drink wine until I was in my forties. I looked on as kids in my class fell victim to the world of drugs but as I observed them, I can honestly say that marijuana was not the gateway for them but in actuality it was ALCOHOL. This is not a judgment against alcohol but merely an observation. Reefer madness from the 1930's had sufficiently terrified the good God fearing Christian folk into avoiding the "demon drug" that would lead to debauchery and delinquency in our youth. President Nixon used racial slurs saying it would "ruin our good white kids". I once announced to my husband in my thirties that I was curious about the effects of marijuana and would probably just try it to see what it was like when I was eighty and by then no one would really care, I wouldn't risk a felony or losing my medical license or going to jail for a curious diversion.

The years past and I continued to join the "war on weed" and judge and belittle hippy, pot smoking "losers" that clearly had no motivation or determination to be contributors to society in any significant way. I avoided parties and chose to study instead.

Then a strange thing happened in medical school. I realized that my ideals as a healer were quickly squelched by money mongering pharmaceutical companies. I was told by a very respected attending physician professor one day when I was markedly stressed over the barrage of information required to memorize and process that 'I needn't worry my pretty little head, too much and just memorize a few medications for blood pressure, antibiotics and the like and I'd make a good living'. At first I was relieved and then I got angry. What the Hell was he saying or thinking? But little did I know how true that would become a reality for the world I was entering. The world where doctors prescribe billions of pharmaceuticals every year and practice what I would call "lazy medicine". What happened to the art of diagnosing and finding the source of the problem? We just funnel patients through like cattle. Seeing on average forty to sixty patients in a day and rolling out those medication prescriptions like glorified legal drug dealers. We are wined and dined by pretty little drug reps and when they could no longer buy us with their expensive gifts, like Caribbean cruises, golf trips, Rolex watches or Mont Blanc pens, they began to use fear tactics to scare us into C.Y.A. medicine (cover your butt, lol). Telling us that if patients are prescribed certain medications we could be sued or liable for their deaths, yet the CDC reports that over 100,000 patients a year die from these medications AS PRESCRIBED. Yes, that's not even overdoses or patients abuse, but as prescribed they cause significant deaths. If 100,000 people died in a bombing or natural disaster we'd be calling in troops or Special Forces or something. Calling for government action or intervention. Yet this quiet poison rainfall insidiously on us takes like a thief in the night our loved ones.

But in all this madness one day a pharmaceutical rep talked to our residency group about Marinol. A synthetic expensive version of THC, the active ingredient in cannabis that is known to be what is called psychoactive or "catnip for humans". It was an acceptable prescription choice, legal and a perfectly good option for patients that were dying anyway, who would not be likely to care about addiction that could treat intractable nausea (most likely from the poisons of the chemotherapy they were imparting) or cachexia (wasting syndrome associated with weight loss and loss of appetite). So with this information and the assurance that it was acceptable and more importantly legal I began prescribing this when indicated but often patients could not afford it at almost $300-$1000 per month even with insurance. So for almost twenty years I have known of the benefits and sharing them with patients. What I didn't know is that the plant is diverse in its healing, anti-cancer, anti-disease, symptom alleviating and psychological impairment treatment potentials.

One of my motivating factors for going into medicine was my sick and ailing father who had intractable grand mal seizures his whole life. Sometimes varying from three a day to thousands a day with intractable status epiliepticus episodes where he was at risk of death. The seizure medications were not only ineffective but eventually, I believe caused his cancer (a rare form of lymphoma known to be caused by these medications) and had we known about the benefits of cannabis might have made a tremendous difference for us. The funny thing was that it was probably right under his nose with hippy older brother back in the seventies and he didn't even know it. We clearly know more about certain strains however and just smoking whatever my brother had may or may not have helped his seizures. It is only through the research and understanding of the different properties of the plant that we can find matches to all sorts of diseases and symptoms that need alleviated. The sad thing is that fear and fiction have muddied the waters and clouded the lens that we are able to see through and see the benefits of the different aspects of the plant. We have not had the opportunities but for those that were willing to risk getting in trouble to come to understand through the veil of hypocrisy, judgment and limited thinking. We have looked to the pharmaceutical companies, the amazon and treated with poisons (chemo), radiation and surgery (necessary and unnecessarily) for solutions and alleviations of many unsolvable predicaments without solution. Thus has come through much education, empowerment and knowing the facts what we call endearingly in this book,

…. THE CANNABIS SOLUTION!

Journey with us as we dispel the myths and uncover the properties that could change the way we view our approach to medicine in the future.

As I began to understand the internal cannabinoid system within the human body, I had a whole new clear understanding of the possibilities of this plant in our modern society.

My personal story is that I began having many health issues as a child. Chronic fatigue, arthritis, headaches and abdominal complaints. All of which I attribute to poor eating habits, lack of good nutrition and extreme stress in our home with my father's illnesses. I thought it was normal to hurt. Normal to live with constant headaches and abdominal pain. Normal to have menstrual cycles that lasted two weeks with hormonal fluctuations that caused many female emotional flares. Normal to feel tired. I wanted so much for my life. My ambitions were stifled by my pain and fatigue so often. I one day made a decision to change my diet and that's how I got through medical school and residency but continued to struggle with hormone issues and had to seek alternative healers to help me understand the way the human body works and how to utilize available options in our environment that God gave us. I learned about natural hormone therapy and it changed my life. The interesting thing is and what I'm about to say is VERY important is that just like you have hormones in your body that drive every process and you can take an external plant natural source of hormones, the body also has a cannabinoid system internally that drives almost every process in your body along side the hormones and you can take an external plant based natural cannabinoid too! Cannabinoids just happen to be found in many plants including Cannabis or what we call Marijuana. So you see any judgments that I had against Marijuana were just fear based and propaganda. That started my journey to understanding what all else I didn't know and opening the door to healing and helping through more than just alternative hormones, nutritional therapy, exercise and stress reduction. Now I have a whole new set of tools in my toolbox or "little black bag" that I can use to help heal and alleviate suffering.

THE CANNABIS SOLUTION.

Chapter 1

Fear Over Facts? & Cannabis Myths

"The illegality of cannabis is outrageous, an impediment to full utilization of a drug which helps produce the serenity and insight, sensitivity and fellowship so desperately needed in this increasingly mad and dangerous world." -Carl Sagan

Facts are rapidly winning over fear with medical cannabis "the botanical name for and also referred to as Marijuana. Which is now legal in over 20 states in the U.S. We have been using marijuana for healing, spiritual rituals, industry and socially for recreation distraction, creativity and inspiration of ideas for since the dawning of our human history dated even back as early as 8000 BC.

There are thousands of peer reviewed journal articles from leading medical institutions that show the medicinal benefits of the cannabis plant of which cannabinoids are derived that can effectively treat symptoms of AIDS, cancer, glaucoma, multiple sclerosis, chronic pain, inflammation, headaches, seizures, trauma and psychological mood disorders and more.

We now know that the cannabinoid system is responsible for endocannabinoid (meaning our own internal human cannabinoid system) regulation of our autonomic nervous system, immune system (Echinacea known to treat and prevent colds has cannabinoids), gastrointestinal tract, appetite, reproductive hormones, cardiovascular health and so much more.

This book is intended to help you understand why this plant has been demonized and how to understand it's properties, remove the stigma associated and blast through the myths of cannabis as a potential source of alleviating pain and suffering in our society.

The term "Cannabis" and "marijuana" are both used when referring to the dried flowers, leaves or stems of the female Cannabis plant. There are over 200 slang terms that refer to this including Mary Jane, pot, weed, grass, Ganga and many others.

The word marijuana was thought to come from the Aztec population of Mexico and came into the English Oxford dictionary in the late 19th century.

What is it?

Okay some nerdy science…. Here we go.

Cannabis pronounced (Can-uh-bus) (/'kaenebis/) is a plant genus considered as having three distinct strains. It has 483 known compounds, only one of which is psychoactive (may change personal perception of the environment) called THC.

1.Cannabis ruderalis

2.Cannabis Indica

3.Cannabis Sativa

These three strains were indigenous to Central and South Asia but are now grown all over the globe. It has been used in multiple industries. It has been used for it's strong fibers, seed, oils and therapeutic properties. The fibers of the Cannabis plant have no psychoactive effect and are referred to as "Hemp" when used for industrial purposes. Hemp is used in paper, textiles, cordage and construction.

Of the 483 compounds, at least 84 are cannabinoids which include THC (tetrahydrocannabivarin), CBN (cannabidiol), CBD (cannabidiol), and CBG (cannabigerol). All with different and specific receptor sites and purposes in the human physiology.

Around 100 million Americans have been estimated to have consumed Cannabis at least once in their lifetime. Despite the strict laws against it, it is estimated over 25 million users regular. The third most common substance behind alcohol and tobacco most likely due last place by its illegality.

The federal illegality still remains an issue despite independent states allowing its use.

The stigma of 'reefer madness' is a serious barrier to the use of the therapeutic understanding of the plant and it's possibilities.

So much of what our concerns are, are based in fear and lack of true knowledge. Myths perpetuated and unfounded. I'm reminded of a story I heard once about a woman who made her family a roast every Sunday. She always lopped off the end of the rump roast and cooked it accordingly, predictably. Appreciated and loved as a staple in their home for Sunday dinner. Never questioned just a tradition. Then one day her husband asked her, "honey, why do you always lop of the end of the roast?" To which her reply was. "Hmmm. You know… I just don't know."

Out of curiosity she called her mother who had taught her to prepare the roast since she was a young girl. She asked her the question her husband had posed to which her reply was, "Hmmm. Because that's the way your grandmother taught me to do it."

Perplexed and curious she then called her grandmother to which her grandmother's response was "well dear, because my pan was too small!"

How often we carry on traditions just because of some reason that we are no longer constrained by or have any effect on us… just because that's the way it has always been done.

We operate out of fear and control for that same reason in many areas of our lives. Just because someone said it, doesn't necessarily make it so. We live our lives from the social and historical experience, not even evidence, that says it's so.

We hear that someone once got "high" and did something crazy. Do we stop to ask if they might have been under the influence of alcohol or other drugs, or that they may have done something crazy anyway? Do we stop to ask if that's even really true? Do we seek to understand all the contributing factors? Do we just assume? How many judgments and assumptions have you lived out in your lifetime based on social and historical experience, not even your own.

So many people have been denied treatment based on this fear. I think about how different my father's life may have been if he had had access to the strains that treat seizures so effectively. Instead of the medications that he took that were not only ineffective but made his personality angry and moody, caused him fatigue and eventually cancer. I wonder if the stigma then would have kept him from getting help that could have helped him based on fear.

The good news is the fear is abating. According to a recent Gallup poll, found that for the first time in the history of the United States, 58% of Americans support legalization of Cannabis.

Lets look at some of the myths

1. Myth: Marijuana can kill you

Fact: There is no lethal dose of Cannabis. Well actually that might not necessarily be true, the lethal dose is impossible to consume, estimated at over 15,000 pounds in a time frame of 15 minutes.

While you can "overdose" based on the definition of "taking more than the normal or recommended dose resulting in untoward effects", when consumed by itself (not with other drugs or alcohol) there is no lethal dose possible to consume.

 2. Myth: Weed will make you a criminal

Fact: There has never been a link between cannabis and violent crime or crimes against property. A recent study, from data from 1990-2006, RG Morris, et al, The effect of Medical Marijuana Laws on Crime, found that higher crime rates are not associated with marijuana.

3. Myth: Marijuana is a gateway drug

Fact: Wisconsin Governor Scott Walker first used the term "Gateway effect" in an interview discussing Wisconsin sheriffs talking about meth and heroin increases. While most of the heavy narcotic, or heroin, meth or heavy drug users have tried marijuana at some point it does not prove that using it leads to harder drug use. More likely is that alcohol abuse is the gateway. Some people are just more prone to addictions and mind-altering drugs. In a recent survey by Nation Institute on Drug Abuse found that marijuana use has increased but heroin, cocaine and methamphetamine use has decreased which would go against the gateway theory.

4. Myth: Cannabis Prohibition protects kids

Fact: Use of marijuana in teenagers hit a peak in 2011 with one out of every 15 high school students reporting use (according to CDC report), but teenagers don't smoke any more in states where medical marijuana is legal than in states where it is not. Some legalization advocates claim that the best way to reduce use by minors is to legalize and regulate dispensaries, reducing the black market power.

5. Myth: Marijuana makes you lazy or lack motivation

Fact: "Amotivational syndrome" has been identified in 5-6% of the population and have difficulties with motivation but has not been associated with Marijuana use. Yes there are lazy Cannabis users, but there are lazy non-cannabis users and successful creative influential cannabis users as well. Of those that have admitted to Cannabis use are, our president Barack Obama, Oprah, Stephen Colbert, Clarence Thomas, Jay-Z. None of these famous people would be considered lazy or lacking in motivation. There is plenty of evidence to the contrary that marijuana can lead to creative and artistic influence than laziness.

6. Myth: Marijuana influence driving "stoned driving" is as bad as "drunk driving"

Fact: Drunk driving kills 28 people per day in America according to studies done by MADD (mother's against drunk driving) and there is no evidence reported for accidents on Cannabis use alone (not commixed with alcohol or other drugs). While Marijuana can affect driving ability users tend to be more cautious and slower drivers reducing accidents.

7. Myth: Supporting Marijuana will help drug dealers and cartels

Fact: Legalizing marijuana in the United States would weaken drug cartels and thus save lives potentially. Estimates put marijuana at 30-50% of drug cartel revenue. Legal dispensaries in the united states would essential divert from this market and thus reduce their ability to control and terrorize by decreasing their financial power. Illegal drug dealers in the United States would not be able to sell to school children as easily if they don't have a market share. While education is needed to prevent diversion within the home there are definite advantages to making it available without the illegal activities associated.

8. Myth: Marijuana causes brain damage

Fact: This has been used by fear mongers for many years on the war on weed. That it causes memory loss and damage. There was a study done in France that lead to this myth based on a very small number of patients, not even significantly significant. It looked at the brains of 20 heavy cannabis users and 20 non-users age 18-25 and while it did show changes related to cognitive and emotional processing, the study authors explained that their results were not conclusive and that they show a correlation with no clear indication whether cannabis changes the brain or whether people with these brain changes were more likely to use or need cannabis for medical indications like brain changes associated with psychological disturbances like Post Traumatic Stress Disorder (PTSD). It is however, known that patients with PTSD are more likely to have a smaller degenerated hippocampus due to chronic trauma and stress. We have no way of knowing if those 20 heavy users age 18-25 were expressed to chemical or emotional stress for example. This study was very small, not statistically significant by most scientific standards and did not look at long-term use and effects of cannabis. If it does change the brain, there is no evidence to say whether those changes are positive or negative.

A study published in 2013 suggests that CBC an cannabinoid specifically found in Marijuana can encourage neurogenesis. A group of researchers tested the effects of adult, mouse neural stem progenitor cells (NSPCs) outside of the body. NSPCs are special types of cells that can differentiate into a variety of other cells, aiding in brain recovery and growth. The team found that CBC increased the viability of these cells, meaning the cannabinoids improved their function.

9. Myth: Marijuana is addictive

Fact: Because we have an internal cannabinoid system, we can no more get addicted to cannabinoids than we can get addicted to other chemicals found in our bodies like hormones or oxygen when taken externally. There was a study done in the 1990's that indicated that 9% of marijuana users become dependent. This study puts marijuana less addictive than it did alcohol at 14% and tobacco at 24%. There is the possibility that this 9% was inflated because the study did not account for marijuana's criminalization. Some measure of the study included things like the amount of time the user spent attempting to acquire the substance, which could be from criminalization not addiction. While the purpose of cannabis can be used to treat medical symptoms and when the cannabis is removed the symptoms return, one could call this a dependence rather than an addiction since addiction implies aberrant activities that imply the criminalization not addiction if not available legally.

10. Myth: All pot smokers look like hippies or delinquents

Fact: While Scooby Doo's friend Shaggy and Cheech and Chong embody the stoner archetype, countless number of Cannabis users do not fit the stereotype. Celebrities like George Clooney, Louis C.K., Bill Maher, Lady Gaga, Jennifer Aniston and Morgan Freeman have spoke out for medicinal uses of Cannabis and not only do not fit the stoner stereo type but are among the most successful, driven, motivated and intelligent productive inspired people in our culture. Since many forms of cannabis have low THC or psychoactive attributes, and are used for medical reasons, the marijuana user that you don't even know about may be your boss, the Mayor or your pastor of your church.

11. Myth: Smoking marijuana is worse for you lungs than cigarettes and can cause cancer

Fact: The main argument against smoking marijuana is that it is smoked without a filter causing more harm that cigarettes and the lungs are not protected.   A 2012 JAMA (Journal of American Medicine) study by Mark J. Pletcher, MD, et al, on Marijuana's effects on the lungs concluded: Occasional and low cumulative marijuana use was not associated with adverse effects on pulmonary function over 20 years. It could be that cigarettes smokers inhale more quantity; there are carcinogens in many common cigarettes today and the fact that Cannabis has medicinal therapeutic and healing qualities.

That said, if your concerned about your lungs there are many ways to consume marijuana besides smoking and many of those forms do not have psychoactive attributes if you are concerned about altering your mood or personality.

As far as cancer is concerned there are hundreds of studies touting the benefits of preventing and not only treating the side effects of cancer drugs but actually reversing or curing cancer. I am not making that claim here, merely supporting numerous studies that do support that claim.

12. Myth: Marijuana turns good kids into troublemakers

Fact: This is definitely a remnant of the "reefer madness" propaganda. A 1990 study (ncbi.nlm.nih.gov Psychosocial correlates of Marijuana use and problem drinking in a National sample of adolescents Richard Jessor, et al) of 10,000 high school juniors and seniors found that marijuana use is only one out of host of unconventional behaviors which correlate with each other. Some adolescents are more rebellious (or independent) than others the these kids are more likely to smoke marijuana or drink alcohol or do other drugs but does not correlate with being the cause.

13. Myth: Doctors believe Marijuana is bad

Fact: The majority of American medical doctors think marijuana should be legal according to a recent study done by WebMD survey reported in April. Cannabis is effective medicine for millions of patients and doctors believe that legalizing would increase access to this powerful medication.

14. Myth: Opposition to legalization of cannabis is driven by cautious prudence

Fact: Oh no no my dear. Pharmaceutical companies (known as big pharma) have everything to gain by keeping medical cannabis out of the hands of patients. While it prudent to be cautious and know the evidence, do your homework and know the facts, the opposition is fueled by industries that figure to lose profits should cannabis become legal and available. Alcohol and big tobacco also stand to lose and believe it or not cotton (which competes with hemp) are all billion-dollar industries that stand to lose in competition. It is easier to pay lobbyists and lawmakers/politicians than to face losing billions of dollars.

I found out that it is not only completely legal to pay lobbyist and politicians for political outcomes but is customary and usual.

15. Myth: Cannabis will make me gain weight because it causes the "Munchies"

Fact: Cannabis consumers reportedly have lower body mass indexes (BMI) and smaller waistlines than non-consumers.

Additional evidence suggests that cannabis consumers are more active, have a lower risk of type 2 diabetes, and 16 percent lower fasting insulin levels. Cannabis consumers are also less likely to be obese. In fact, a 2011 study found that regular cannabis consumption was associated with reduced obesity rates by roughly one-third.

A study done in 2015, found that tetrahydrocannabinol (THC) treatment reduced weight gain, fat gain, and energy intake in obese mice. THC is the chemical compound that causes the famous cannabis "high." The rodents had become obese after being given foods that caused them to gain weight. The mice were treated with THC daily for three weeks and the dosage of cannabinoid was increased on the fourth week. Luckily, the compound inspired weight loss in obese mice, it did not cause weight loss in mice that were already lean.

Of interest also, Canadian scientists studied the intestinal microbes of the mice. Inside the gut lives up to 4.4 pounds of live microorganisms. These microorganisms work synergistically with cells in the digestive tract to break down foods, maintain good health, and can promote weight loss or weight gain. It has been shown that overweight people and thin people have different gut bacteria. Very important to know if you want to lose weight, FYI. The study found that THC caused changes in the gut microbiome that are thought to contribute to healthy weight. Specifically, the psychoactive changed the ratio of weight-promoting microbes in the digestive tract to a healthier balance after being fed a high-fat diet. While amazing, this action is not entirely surprising. It is well-known that THC has powerful antimicrobial qualities and is thought to protect the cannabis plant from pathogenic infections. THC is not the only cannabis compound that is expected to encourage weight loss. Research has shown that cannabidiol (CBD), a cannabinoid that does not cause a high, can block some of THC's effect on appetite. Additional research shows that CBD can reduce appetite and feeding time in rodents. Research in the field of obesity and diabetes suggests that the cannabis compound tetrahydrocannabivarin (THCV) may also promote weight loss in rodents as well as balance blood sugar, reduce inflammation of the pancreas, and improve insulin sensitivity. Of course, simply smoking cannabis is not the only factor that may contribute to weight loss. Physical exercise, a balanced diet, adequate sleep, stress reduction, and pleasurable social activities all promote good health and lend a hand in weight management.

THC binds to receptor cells in the brain that trigger a hormone called Ghrelin (hormone that triggers hunger) and the higher the THC content the more the hunger is triggered acutely. However there are cannabinoids that are known to decrease appetite or work antagonistically or trigger leptin (the hormone that triggers fullness) and those cannabinoids are CBD (cannabidiol), CBN (cannabinol) and CBG (cannabigerol) as well as THCv which not only triggers leptin but improves insulin resistance (hormone that can cause weight gain).

Study done in 2011, American Journal of epidemiology showed weight loss in regular users and a study done by the American Journal of Medicine with over 14,000 adults showed a 16% lower insulin, and 17% lower insulin resistance with a smaller waist circumference.

There is also an anti-inflammatory effect with CBD which studies have shown inflammation linked to obesity and obesity related disease. A study done in 2003 showed that

CBD also activated the endocannabinoid system in exercise related metabolism and and showed decreased obesity rates lower for regular cannabis users due to adaptive down regulation of endocannabinoid signaling with long term dampening of CB1 receptors. There was a pharmaceutical developed in Europe called "Accomplia" that used these cannabinoids to aid in weight loss. It has also been shown that THCv increases metabolism and it has been also shown that the top 6 healthiest states in America have legalized Cannabis.

Myth 16: Cannabis may make you eat more sugar and worsen diabetes.

Fact: Diabetes type 1 has been shown to be an autoimmune disorder that is triggered by leaky gut and inflammation. Type 2 is well known to be due to insulin resistance. Both which are improved by multiple cannabinoids. Stimulation of CB1 receptors have been shown to stabilize blood sugar, work as anti-inflammatory, are neuroprotective (essential in diabetic neuropathy and diabetic brain related disease (like Alzheimer's), anti-spasmodic (muscle relaxer in the gut for issues like diabetic gastropathy or slow digestion related to diabetes), improve sleep and restless leg syndrome, decrease cholesterol, lower stress (through the lowering cortisol the stress hormone), improve retinopathy (eye disease related to increased pressure and inflammation) and decrease gluconeogenesis (production of sugar by the liver, hormonally mediated in diabetes).

A study done in 2001 shoed that mice given THC in high amounts (150 mg/kg) had decreased hyperglycemia (high blood sugar), decreased pancreatic insulin resistance and decreased inflammation markers. A study done in 2012 showed that CBD showed decreased feeding in rats and CBD showed rats to have decreased appetite, less metabolic fatty liver disease and THCv showed decrease in glucose intolerance, increase in insulin sensitivity and increased energy expenditure. CBG showed no effect on appetite. 2015 study showed a decrease in neuropathic pain and decreased retinopathy (eye disease).

One by one these myths fall away and only the truth is left. So why did these myths become so prevalent and widespread. Lets talk about the history….

Chapter 2

History

As the myths fall away we are seeing more laws based on science and common sense, peer reviewed evidence based information and a focus on public health interventions rather than propaganda. Since Cannabis was criminalized in the 1930's we have seen a lot of changes. Currently about 750,000 people are arrested each year for marijuana offenses in the United States. Not all arrests lead to prosecution and few people prosecute and convicted of simple possession end up in jail. Most are fined or place into community supervision. About 40,000 inmates of state and federal prison have a current conviction involving marijuana and about half of them are in for marijuana offense alone. Most are involved in distribution. This has lead to tremendous cost to the taxpayers and not decreased marijuana usage at all. In fact it has increased in usage. Partly due to the knowledge of growing different strains for different uses. In the past if you wanted to try marijuana for a specific purpose you just bought off the street and that may help your symptoms or that particular strain based on the THC to cannabinoid ratio may make you better or worse. Despite the glorification in pop culture, many federal prisons are still packed with non-violent marijuana offenders.

While some do hard time, some openly flaunt usage in legalized states like California in music festivals like Coachella (colloquial for Cannabis) and celebrate the counterculture.

Often, unfortunately marijuana is a drug that has been vilified for various reasons and mostly has it's roots in race and social class associations.

In the 17ᵗʰ century hemp was actively used to make rope and fabric. In the 19ᵗʰ century cannabis was used as a popular ingredient in many medications.

Hashish became a fad used in upper middle class society, with higher concentrations of the psychotropic effect of THC (see chapter on Cannabis 101 for details about THC to cannabinoid ratios and effects).

Hundreds of Hashis Parlors popped up in New York along with opium dens.

When did marijuana become well known to the average to lower class? When there was a large wave of immigration from Mexico in the early 1900s. They brought with them the societal tradition of recreational smoking of marijuana much like the American Indians with peace pipes and Peyote practices. It was first marihuana and was often misspelled by Americans. Resentment towards these immigrants, scarcity mentality of lost jobs but more aggressive work force and soon after the American war of 1898, anti-drug campaigners realized they could use this societal connection to their advantage. The resentment grew into the 1930's when The Great Depression marked rampant unemployment. Fear of scarcity and losing jobs was exploited by the anti-drug propagandists for obvious reason.

Thus brought in the father of the "War on Weed", Harry J. Anslinger, Federal Bureau of Narcotics commissioner when he launched a campaign against marijuana. He claimed that marijuana or marihuana called at the time made Mexicans dangerous. Bogus research was produced to back up these claims and the war on weed was fueled with fire of anti-racial slurs and claims.

The Mexican culture was under fire and the presumed demonization was underway by attacking aspects of their culture that could easily be targeted. After the Federal Bureau of Narcotics was created in 1930 marijuana was illegal in 29 states by 1931. In 1936 the propaganda film "Reefer Madness" did exactly what it was supposed to do: create panic and fear. The Marijuana tax act in 1937 officially criminalized unauthorized possession. The US tobacco industry was booming and the legislature began to grow teeth against this supposed demon. Laws in the 1950s created mandatory sentencing for drug related crimes but repealed by the 70s when they appeared to have no affect on usage of marijuana.

President Richard Nixon using the war on weed to attach his enemies. It wasn't legal to discriminate but associating Mexicans, hippies and African Americans with drugs, they could criminalize all heavily. They could arrest their leaders, raid homes, and break up meetings with a purpose, it was reported to Harper's magazine by former domestic policy chief John Ehrlichman.

Congress passed the Controlled substances act in 1970 and made marijuana a Schedule 1 substance, which this category indicates that it is illegal with no approved medical purposes. It was intended to be only temporary until further research could be done. Congress acknowledged that they didn't know enough about the substance to make any long-term conclusions about its potential uses. Nixon continuing his efforts to use the attack for political gain created a committee that was committed to targeting racial profiles for criminalization. He appointed nine commissioners with an evident agenda. They launched fifty research projects, polled the public and members of the justice community and took thousands of pages of testimony. The committee after the research came out could not deny the potential medicinal effects of marijuana and started talk of legalization. When Nixon heard about this he denounced the commission, just months before they were to issue their reports.

The commissioner tried to negotiate with Nixon, saying that they would not fight for legalization but to demystify it as a potential medicine and debunk marijuana propaganda. Ultimately they found that marijuana did not cause crime or aggression, lead to harder drug use or cause biochemical or mental or psychological abnormalities. His report ultimately stated that "Marihuana's relative potential for harm to the vast majority of individuals users and its actual impact on society does not justify a social policy designed to seek out and firmly punish those who use it."

Nixon refused to hear the reports and demoted the team. He saw marijuana as tied to "radical demonstrators" and that "Jewish psychiatrists were behind the advocacy for legalizations, when they touted the benefits for what we now label as PTSD related to concentration camps. Problem was that Jewish shop owners were being targeted for taxation what we would now days call dispensaries. He was quoted as saying, "people use marijuana to get high and alcohol to have fun". And he was recorded in later revealed tapes saying to Bo Haldeman, an advisor, "What the Christ is the matter with the Jews, Bob?" referring to their disproportionate use of marijuana. He also claimed that Communists were using it as a weapon. He was also quoted saying, "homosexuality, dope, immorality in general are the enemies of strong societies." And "enforce the law, you've got to scare them."

Marijuana arrests jumped to over 400,000 that year he made those comments. Since then nearly 15 million people have been arrested for marijuana offenses.

For 30 years the U.S. has taken the path of Nixon's prejudice and ignored the experts.

The 1980's brought the Reagan administration that fueled the war on weed with more racial profiling of the drug, demonizing it further and causing more fear and concern.

Fast forward to today from Donald Trump's campaign about Mexican immigrants. Donald Trump was quoted as saying regarding Mexicans, "They're brining drugs. They're bringing crime."

The war is certainly not over. With nearly half of all inmates in American prisons are there for drug related charges and 27% for marijuana related charges, we have many discrepancies in what we believe going forward and the implications of legalization and how would that affect those already in the prison system. At first glance it looks like they are using taxpayer resources but then there is the aspect that many prisons are 'for profit' and have much to gain by low risk criminals.

A new study by UC-Berkley found that prisons are filled with racial disparities. The sentencing project estimated that 1 in 3 black men will spend time behind bars at one time in their life, compared with 1 in 17 white men. Marijuana arrest rates arrest rates are four times higher for black men than white and black men spend an average of 20% more time behind bars than white peers in federal prison.

Private prisons house over 125,000 inmates for the federal government since 2010 with private companies like CEO or Corrections Corp. of America in states like California, Arizona and Texas. It has been found that private facilities house higher percentages of prisoners with low care costs or exclude people with high medial care costs from their contracts.

Young healthy inmates have come into the system since the war on drugs went into effect and disproportionately of color. Private prisons make money and it's all about how they can make the most, highest profit margins with lowest cost.

So, make your conclusions. Consider who is to gain by demonizing Cannabis. Consider who is to gain by legalizing it for medical purposes. But before you make your conclusions let me share with you the properties of this amazing plant. Lets go back to the drawing board and talk about what Medical Cannabis is and what it can do.

Chapter 3

Medical Cannabis 101

The first thing that you need to know is that we all have something called the endocannabinoid system ECS is a group of endogenous cannabinoid receptors located in the mammalian brain and throughout the central and peripheral nervous system that affect homeostasis or regulation of all chemical processes in the body.

 Including but not limited to the immune system, appetite, sleep/wake, mood and hormone balance.

 Have you ever wondered why we are all affected so differently by marijuana? Why the first time you use it, nothing appears to happen? Why some get sleepy, some paranoid, some feel no pain, and some have heightened sensitivities? Some have elevated creativity and focus and some feel 'stoned' and sleepy? Why some love it and some hate it?

Well all of this can be explained through something called the endocannabinoid system, which was first discovered in 1992 by a nerdy scientist Raphael Mechoulam and NIMH researchers William Devane and Dr. Lumir Hanus. Anandamide was the first naturally occurring endogenous (means found within the body) cannabinoid or endocannabinoid.

What you are about to learn next if you don't already know it is that those differences make the diverse healing and health properties of the plant.

Only in the last couple of decades have researchers actually understood what makes the plant and it's strains so diverse and amazing in it's properties.

In 1964 a scientist from Israel named Raphael Mechoulam identified and isolated THC (tetrahydrocannabinol) for the first time and then CBD as well.

Isolating these cannabinoids was the first step to identifying the endocannabinoid system- a biological system of immense importance.

1988 a poor little rat revealed his cannabinoid receptors to these scientists, more prevalent than any other neurotransmitter receptor in the brain. Researchers then began mimicking and producing synthetic versions of THC that could alleviate nausea and wasting syndrome in patients from cancer or HIV. (Now FDA approved called Marinol and prescribed medically by doctors for over thirty years. They started mapping these receptors and found them in regions of the brain that control memory, higher thinking, motor coordination, appetite, immune function, and emotional processing among many.

In 1990 Lisa Matsuda announce at the National Academy of Science's institute of Medicine that she and her colleagues had found the DNA sequence that defined a THC-sensitive receptor in another poor little rat's brain.

They soon cloned that receptor, that would allow them to deactivate receptors (meaning no effect from THC), then since the chemical had no where to latch on to or bind, there was no way to trigger psychoactive behavior (what I commonly refer to as 'cat nip' for humans behavior) or what is commonly referred to as getting high with sativa strains or stoned with indica strains.

This proved that THC worked in the receptors in the brain and central nervous system called CB1.

In 1993 a second receptor was found in the immune and central nervous system called CB2 and these were found plentiful in the gut, spleen, liver, blood vessels, kidneys, bones, lymph cells and reproductive organs.

So, researchers had the receptors now they had to identify the molecules that these receptors received. In 1992, the first endocannabinoid was discovered and named Anadamide (Sanskrit word for 'bliss').

So just like you have hormones in your body and you can take plant-based hormones, you have endocannabinoids but can take plant-based cannabinoids. Within your body it's called endogenous cannabinoids or endocannabinoids or plant based called exogenous cannabinoids.

The second endocannabinoid, found in 1995, was named 2-arachidonoylgycerol or "2-AG" and attached to CB1 and CB2 receptors.

Since then we have discovered that endocannabinoid system is responsible for processes in our body that we are yet even to discover. Possibilities range from treating or preventing cancer to maintaining bone density and hormone balance or mood balance.

The possibilities are endless. Research has shown that small doses of plant cannabinoids from Cannabis can signal the body to make more endocannabinoids and build more receptors.

The first time you use Cannabis you may not feel any affect at all for this reason but by the second or third time they take external cannabinoids can up regulate their receptors (CB1 or CB2… and research is now looking for a third CB3) which are then ready to respond and regulate multiple chemical processes in the body. Unlike drugs that require more and more to get the same effect like methamphetamines or cocaine needed in larger amounts to produce the same dopamine (brain chemical) response, Cannabis requires less by up regulating receptors making aberrant drug seeking behaviors requiring more drug for desired effect a non-issue. More receptors increase a person's sensitivities and smaller doses have larger effects and enhanced baseline of activity.

Isn't it ironic that we all have this system within us and we didn't even know it? That we judge the plant based on propaganda and not science or truth. That we all have cannabinoids floating around in us every second and have yet to understand the gift of the Ganga. Lol.

Chapter 4

Conditions Treated

As you can see there are various receptors and for all these receptors there are cannabinoids, endogenous or exogenous that turn them on or off in all the systems of all animals including humans. So lets look at some of the conditions that can be treated, which is probably all disease or out of balance systems that need alignment to occur to be whole and well.

If you understand the endocannabinoids then you can begin to understand how we might use plant-based cannabinoids to treat imbalances.

What makes cannabinoids medicine? Understanding what cannabinoids are is essential here. Cannabinoids are compounds secreted by the Cannabis plant flowers work their magic by mimicking compounds our bodies naturally produce called endocannabinoids and mediate chemical communication between cells, fill in deficient messaging and regulate missing messaging which create disease and untoward symptoms of disease.

When Cannabis is consumed, cannabinoids bind to receptor sites (CB1 or CB2) throughout the body and respond diversely depending on amounts and types.

THC binds to receptors in the brain (CB1) where as CBN (cannabinol) binds with affinity to CB2 receptors through out the body. Depending on different hybrid strains grown more or less of THC or Cannabinol can be accentuated for different receptors and purposes.

The following are the conditions that can be treated with medical

Cannabis:

- Acquired Hypothyroidism
- Acute Gastritis
- Agoraphobia
- AIDS Related Illness
- Alcohol Abuse
- Alcoholism
- Alopecia Areata
- Alzheimer's Disease
- Amphetamine Dependency
- Amyloidosis
- Amyotrophic Lateral Sclerosis (ALS)
- Angina Pectoris
- Ankylosis
- Anorexia
- Anorexia Nervosa
- Anxiety Disorders
- Any Chronic Medical Symptom that Limits Major Life Activities
- Arachnoiditis
- Arnold-Chiari Malformation
- Arteriosclerotic Heart Disease
- Arthritis
- Arthropathy, gout
- Asthma
- Attention Deficit Hyperactivity Disorder (ADD/ADHD)
- Auditory Neuropathy
- Autism/Aspergers
- Autoimmune Disease
- Autonomic Neuropathy
- Back Pain
- Back Sprain
- Bell's Palsy
- Bipolar Disorder
- Brain Tumor, Malignant
- Bruxism
- Bulimia
- Cachexia
- Cancer
- Cancer, Adrenal Cortical
- Cancer, Endometrial
- Cancer, Prostate
- Cancer, Testicular
- Cancer, Uterine
- Carpal Tunnel Syndrome
- Causalgia
- Cerebral Palsy
- Cervical Disk Disease
- Cervicobrachial Syndrome
- Chemotherapy
- Chemotherapy Induced Anorexia
- Chronic Fatigue Syndrome

- Chronic Inflammatory Demyelinating Polyneuropathy
- Chronic Migraine
- Chronic Pain
- Chronic Pancreatitis
- Chronic renal failure
- Chronic Traumatic Encephalopathy
- Cocaine Dependence
- Colitis
- collagenous colitis
- Conjunctivitis
- Constipation
- Cranial Neuropathy
- Crohn's Disease
- CRPS (Complex Regional Pain Syndrome Type II)
- Cystic Fibrosis
- Darier's Disease
- Decompensated Cirrhosis
- Degenerative Arthritis
- Degenerative Arthropathy
- Delirium Tremens
- Dermatomyositis
- Diabetes, Adult Onset
- Diabetes, Insulin Dependent
- Diabetic Neuropathy
- Diabetic Peripheral Vascular Disease
- Diarrhea
- Diverticulitis
- Dysthymic Disorder
- Dystonia
- Eczema
- Elevated Intraocular Pressure
- Emphysema
- Endometriosis
- Epidermolysis Bullosa
- Epididymitis
- Epilepsy
- Failed Back Surgery Syndrome with reoccurring back pain
- Felty's Syndrome
- Fibromyalgia
- Fibrous Dysplasia
- Focal Neuropathy
- Friedreich's Ataxia
- Gastritis
- Genital Herpes
- Glaucoma
- Glioblastoma Multiforme
- Graves Disease
- Headaches, Cluster
- Headaches, Tension
- Hemophilia A
- Henoch-Schonlein Purpura
- Hepatitis C

- Hepatitis C currently receiving antiviral treatment
- Hereditary Spinal Ataxia
- HIV/AIDS
- Hospice Patients
- Huntington's Disease
- Hydrocephalus
- Hydromyelia
- Hypertension
- Hyperventilation
- Hypoglycemia
- Impotence
- Inflammatory autoimmune-mediated arthritis
- Inflammatory Bowel Disease (IBD)
- Insomnia
- Intermittent Explosive Disorder (IED)
- Interstitial Cystitis
- Irritable Bowel Syndrome
- Lipomatosis
- Lou Gehrig's Disease
- Lupus
- Lyme Disease
- lymphocytic colits
- Lymphoma
- Major Depression
- Malignant Melanoma
- Mania
- Melorheostosis
- Meniere's Disease
- Mitochondrial disease
- Motion Sickness
- Mucopolysaccharidosis (MPS)
- Multiple Sclerosis (MS)
- Muscle Spasms
- Muscular Dystrophy
- Myasthenia Gravis
- Myeloid Leukemia
- Myoclonus
- Nail-Patella Syndrome
- Neurofibromatosis
- Neuropathy
- Nightmares
- Obesity
- Obsessive Compulsive Disorder
- One or more injuries that significantly interferes with daily activities as documented by the patient's provider
- Opiate Dependence
- Optic Neuropathy
- Osteoarthritis
- Panic Disorder
- Parkinson's Disease
- Peripheral Neuropathy
- Peritoneal Pain

- Porphyria
- Post Concussion Syndrome
- Post Polio Syndrome (PPS)
- Post-Laminectomy Syndrome with chronic radiculopathy
- Post-traumatic arthritis
- Post-Traumatic Stress Disorder (PTSD)
- Post-Traumatic Stress Disorder (PTSD) effective August 1, 2017
- Premenstrual Syndrome (PMS)
- Prostatitis
- Psoriatic Arthritis
- Pulmonary Fibrosis
- Quadriplegia
- Radiation Therapy
- Raynaud's Disease
- Reflex Sympathetic Dystrophy
- Reiter's Syndrome
- Residual Limb Pain
- Restless Legs Syndrome (RLS)
- Rheumatoid Arthritis
- Rosacea
- RSD (Complex Regional Pain Syndrome Type 1)
- Schizoaffective Disorder
- Schizophrenia
- Scoliosis
- Sedative Dependence
- Seizures
- Senile Dementia
- Severe Nausea
- Severe Psoriasis
- Severe Vomiting
- Shingles (Herpes Zoster)
- Sickle Cell Anemia
- Sickle Cell Disease
- Sinusitis
- Sjoren's Syndrome
- Skeletal Muscular Spasticity
- Sleep Apnea
- Sleep Disorders
- Small Fiber Neuropathy
- Spasticity
- Spinal Cord Disease
- Spinal Cord Injury
- Spinal Cord Injury with spasticity
- Spinal Stenosis
- Spinocerebellar Ataxia
- Sturge-Weber Syndrome (SWS)
- Stuttering
- Syringomyelia
- Tardive Dyskinesia (TD)
- Tarlov Cysts
- Temporomandibular joint disorder (TMJ)
- Tenosynovitis

- Terminal Illness
- Thyroiditis
- Tic Douloureux
- Tietze's Syndrome
- Tinnitus
- Tobacco Dependence
- Tourette's Syndrome
- Traumatic Brain Injury
- Trichotillomania
- Ulcerative Colitis
- Viral Hepatitis
- Wasting Syndrome
- Whiplash
- Wittmaack-Ekbom's Syndrome
- Writers' Cramp

As you can see just about any process in the human body that results as something out of balance can be treated or at least they symptoms of the disease treated with medical Cannabis.

The qualifying conditions will vary from state to state. Since I am a physician in Arkansas, I have included the qualifying conditions for Arkansas:

Arkansas

Qualifying conditions for the Arkansas Medical Marijuana Amendment include:

- Cancer
- Glaucoma
- HIV/AIDS
- Hepatitis C
- ALS or Lou Gehrig's Disease
- Tourette's Syndrome
- Crohn's disease
- Ulcerative colitis
- Post-traumatic Stress Disorder (PTSD)
- Severe arthritis
- Fibromyalgia
- Alzheimer's disease
- A chronic or debilitating disease that produces:
- Cachexia or wasting syndrome
- Peripheral neuropathy
- Intractable pain
- Severe nausea
- Seizures, including those characteristic of epilepsy
- Severe or persistent muscle spasms, including those characteristic of multiple sclerosis

For more information, please refer to Issue 6 – The Arkansas Medical Marijuana Act of 2016.

Okay, so you may be thinking. I have one of those conditions. I have the diagnosis made by a physician and now I need to know what to look for to treat that condition or symptom. Most dispensaries will be knowledgeable but you want to be informed so it's good to know what you need to get the best results. You will need a basic understanding of the external or exogenous plant based cannabinoids to get the best results for your condition. Just like taking a plant-based hormone that fits the receptors in your body, there are different cannabinoids that target different receptors for different things.

Here is an explanation of the following most common external or plant based cannabinoids used to treat symptoms or conditions.

THC, CBD, CBN, CBC, CBG and about 80 other chemicals are all in a class of compounds known as cannabinoids, found in abundance in the cannabis plant. Cannabinoids are responsible for many of the effects of cannabis consumption and have important therapeutic benefits.

<u>Delta-9-Tetrahydrocannabinol or (THC)</u> is a psychoactive cannabinoid responsible for many of the effects experienced by the cannabis user. Mild to moderate pain relief, relaxation, insomnia and appetite stimulation. THC has been demonstrated to have anti-depressant effects. The majority of strains range from 12-21% THC with very potent and carefully prepared strains reaching even higher. Average THC potency is about 16-17% in Northern CA. Recent research that suggests patients with a pre-disposition to schizophrenia and anxiety disorders should avoid high-THC cannabis.

Cannabidiol or (CBD) occurs in many strains, at low levels, <1%. In rare cases, CBD can be the dominant cannabinoid, as high as 15% by weight. Popular CBD-rich strains (>4% CBD) include Sour Tsunami, Harlequin and Cannatonic. It can provide relief for chronic pain due to muscle spasticity, convulsions and inflammation. Offering relief for patients with MS, Fibromyalgia and Epilepsy. Some researchers feel it provides effective relief from anxiety-related disorders. CBD has also been shown to inhibit cancer cell growth when injected into breast and brain tumors in combination with THC.

Cannabinol or (CBN) is an oxidative degradation product of THC. It may result from improper storage or curing and extensive processing, such as when making concentrates. It is usually formed when THC is exposed to UV light and oxygen over time. CBN has some psychoactive properties, about 10% of the strength of THC. CBN is thought by researchers to enhance the dizziness and disorientation users of cannabis may experience. It may cause feelings of grogginess and has been shown to reduce heart rate. Cannabichromene or (CBC) is a rare, non-psychoactive cannabinoid, usually found at low levels (<1%) when present. Research conducted has shown CBC has anti-depressant effects, 10x those of CBD. CBC has also been shown to improve the pain-relieving effects of THC. Studies have demonstrated that CBC has sedative effects, promoting relaxation.

Cannabigerol or (CBG) is a non-psychoactive cannabinoid. It is commonly found in cannabis. CBG-acid is the precursor to both THC-acid and CBD-acid in the plant usually found at low levels (<1%) when present. Researchers have demonstrated both pain relieving and inflammation reducing effects. CBG reduces intraocular pressure, associated with glaucoma. CBG has been shown to have antibiotic properties and to inhibit platelet aggregation, which slows the rate of blood clotting.

<u>Cannabichromene or (CBC)</u>

Encourages brain growth. For a long time, it was thought that the brain stops developing once you reach a certain age. Turns out, this is not the case. Cells responsible for memory and learning, for example, are continuously made via a process called neurogenesis. In folks with dementia and Alzheimer's, neurogenesis is altered. A study published in 2013 suggests that CBC can encourage neurogenesis. A group of researchers tested the effects of adult, mouse neural stem progenitor cells (NSPCs) outside of the body. NSPCs are special types of cells that can differentiate into a variety of other cells, aiding in brain recovery and growth. The team found that CBC increased the viability of these cells, meaning the cannabinoids improved their function. Used as an anti-depressant, CBC is a non-psychoactive compound. This means that those looking for medical relief without a high might appreciate CBC as a medical alternative. Though THC and CBD are commonly thought of as antidepressants, research suggests that cannabichromene can also lend a helping hand. Using rodent models, researchers from the University of Mississippi found that rats treated with CBC performed significantly better on stress tests. Chronic stress is considered one of the primary trigger factors for depression. The better you can adapt from stress, the less likely you are to experience depression. As an anti-inflammatory, inflammation is at the root of many modern diseases. While a little inflammation is a healthy immune response, it seems to run rampant in conditions like autoimmune diseases, allergy, and even psychiatric conditions like depression and schizophrenia. A 2010 study found that CBC worked as an anti-inflammatory alone, but its inflammation-busting powers are amplified when combined with THC. The combination of the two cannabinoids was more successful in fighting inflammation than either one of them alone. This little cannabinoid may have a big impact on pain. 2011 research found that CBC and CBD both stimulated pain-reliving networks in animal models. Early research from the 1980s found that CBC again worked with THC to produce potent analgesic effects. The pain-fighting properties of both cannabinoids increased when combined. CBC has mild analgesic properties on its own. As an antibacterial and antifungal, apparently, the 1980s were a hay-day for CBC research. Another early study found that CBC had significant antibacterial properties. The cannabinoid put dreaded E. coli and staph colonies in their place. CBC also had "mild to moderate" anti-fungal properties as well. This information goes hand-in-hand with a more recent study, which found that CBC and other cannabioids were as effective as Vancomycin against MRSA.

Tetrahydrocannabinolic acid or (THCa) is a cannabis compound that is beginning to demonstrate immense therapeutic potential despite the infancy of its research. You've heard of THC, and while they may sound similar, THCa actually has very different properties. Unlike THC, THCa is a non-psychoactive cannabinoid found in raw and live cannabis. As the plant dries, THCa slowly converts to THC. Heat expedites this conversion in a process known as decarboxylation, a fancy word that describes what happens when you smoke or vaporize flower. If you've purchased lab-tested cannabis, you may notice that the most abundant cannabinoid is either THC or THCA, either of which can stretch between 10-20% on average. While THCa is the more accurate label for flower that hasn't been decarboxylated, they essentially mean the same thing if you assume the consumer intends on smoking, vaporizing, or heating the product in some way. There isn't enough research on THCa to definitively state what it can treat and with what degree of efficacy, but preliminary research and anecdotal evidence suggest that THCa will play a pivotal role in cannabis medicine as the industry propels forward. Here are some of the potential benefits studies have started to unveil:

Anti-inflammatory properties for treatment of arthritis and lupus

Neuroprotective properties for treatment of neurodegenerative diseases

Anti-emetic properties for treatment of nausea and appetite loss

Anti-proliferative properties noted in studies of prostate cancer

Other possible medicinal avenues supported by patient stories include insomnia, muscle spasms, and pain

Every high-THC strain that has not yet been decarboxylated contains THCa, and these cannabinoid levels are particularly high as a live or freshly harvested plant. For this reason, raw cannabis parts are popularly juiced for their THCA benefits.

tetrahydrocannabivarin or (THCv) THCv is thought to have some psychoactive potential. Research has shown that in low doses, THCv may reduce the psychoactivity of THC. In high doses, however, it seems to connect to the same locations in the brain and body as traditional THC. Though, more research is needed to clear up these associations. In early tests, THCV has shown about 25 percent the potency of THC. Though more research is needed, it is thought that THCV may be part of what gives strains classified as sativas their quick onset and energizing mental high. It is used as an antioxidant, anti-inflammatory (including experimental inflammation of the gut), Weight loss (there is some evidence from animal trials that pure THCV is an appetite suppressant and may reduce food intake. In a

2007 study presented at the IACM 4th Conference on Cannabinoids in Medicine, researchers found that mice treated with THCV alone spent less time around their food and did not eat as much as other rats.) When THCV is combined with THC, however, rodents did not experience weight loss and did not show a reduction in appetite. Research on other cannabinoids, including cannabidiol (CBD), has shown that some nonpsychoactive cannabinoids may decrease appetite. This promising research suggests that both CBD and THCV may help curb the munchies and promote weight loss. Some indication for Diabetes, in phase 2 clinical trials of 62 patients, researchers at GW Pharmaceuticals tested the effects of CBD and THCV in patients with type 2 diabetes. The trials tested 100mg of CBD and 5mg of THCV. The researchers looked at these compounds alone as well as in a 20:1 ratio.

The trials showed that THCV and CBD successfully improved fasting insulin levels, reduced blood glucose levels, improved insulin response, reduced blood pressure, and reduced inflammation markers. Though these trials are preliminary, this gives the cannabinoids potential value in diabetes treatment. Several different compounds in the cannabis plant have shown powerful effects against seizure and epileptic convulsions. The two most common cannabis compounds for epilepsy are CBD and THC. Now, early research shows that THCV has anti-convulsant properties as well. In rodent models, THCV has successfully quelled seizure activity. Researchers think that this is because of the way THCV engages the nervous system. Similar to psychoactive THC, THCV binds to special cell receptors (the CB1 and CB2 receptor) that may play a role in managing excessive excitement in the brain. An overly excited brain contributes to epilepsy. THCV has also shown promise in animal studies of Parkinson's disease. A 2011 study published in the British Journal of Pharmacology wanted to see if THCV would improve the motor function of rats with an experimental form of Parkinson's disease. THCV can block certain cell receptors that are targeted by THC. In certain doses, THCV decreases the activation of the CB1 receptor. The CB1 receptor is a location on the surface of a cell that contributes to the psychoactive effects of cannabis. While THCV can block the CB1 receptor, it also triggers the CB2 receptor. The CB1 receptor is primarily concentrated in the nervous system, and the CB2 is concentrated in the immune system. Researchers speculated that these unique properties of THCV would make it a particularly useful Parkinson's medication.

Cannabinoids are fascinating chemicals. Not only do they have powerful medicinal qualities as individual compounds, but also they work together synergistically to create more potent effects. Each and every cannabinoid deserves some time in the spotlight. With more research on cannabinoids coming out every year, we'll only continue to unveil the amazing healing powers of the cannabis plant.

Target Cannabinoids for conditions

GI issues
      Appetite loss – THC
      Anorexia/Wasting/Nausea – THC/CBD
      Diabetes- CBD/THCV
      Chron's- CBD/THC/THCa
Mood/Behavior
      Anxiety- CBD/CBG
      ADD/ADHD-CBD/THC
      Stress-CBD/THC
      Bipolar-CBD/CBG/THC
      OCD-CBD/CBG/THC
      PTSD-CBD/CBG/THC
      Depression- CBC/CBD/CBG/CBN/THC
Neurological
      Tourettes-THC

Epilepsy/Seizures-CBD/CBN/THCa/THCV
MS- CBD/CBN/THC/THCa
Alzheimers-CBC/CBD/CBG/THC/THCa
Parkinson's-CBC/CBD/CBG/THC/THCa
Spacticity/Muscle Spasms-CBD/CBG/CBN/THC/THCa
Osteoporosis-CBC/CBD/CBG/CBN/THCa
ALS-CBC/CBD/CBG/CBN/THC/THCa

Other

Asthma-THC
Fatigue-THC
High Blood Pressure-CBD/THC
Glaucoma-CBG/THC
HIV/AIDS-THC/THCa
Muscular Dystrophy-CBC/CBD/CBG/THC
Cancer-CBC/CBD/CBDa/CBG/THC/THCa

Pain/Sleep

Sleep Apnea-THC
Cramps-CBD/THC
Migraine/Headache-CBD/THC
Phantom Limb Pain-CBD/THC
Spinal Injury-CBD/THC
Fibromyalgia-CBD/CBN/THC
Insomnia-CBC/CBD/CBN/THC
Chronic Pain-CBC/CBD/CBN/CBG/CBN/THC/THCa
Arthritis/Inflammation-
CBC/CBD/CBDa/CBG/CBN/THC/THCa

Chapter 5

Strains as Medicine

To start, look at the strains as if they are on a spectrum. On one side, there are Indica strains, which tend to be very relaxing and soporific. On the other end, there are Sativas, which increase energy and alertness.

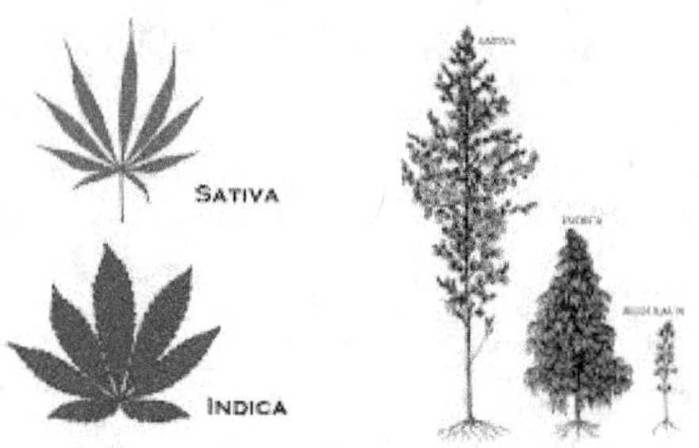

Indica -----------------------Hybrid---------------------Sativa

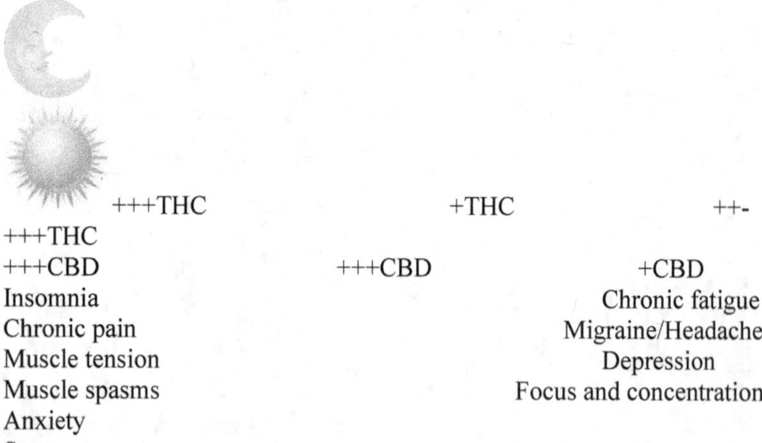

	+++THC	+THC	++-
+++THC			
+++CBD	+++CBD	+CBD	
Insomnia		Chronic fatigue	
Chronic pain		Migraine/Headache	
Muscle tension		Depression	
Muscle spasms		Focus and concentration	
Anxiety			
Stress			

Depending on your desired experience, you can choose your strain based on where it falls between the two (which is often indicated in the form of a percentage).

Of course, it isn't really that simple. Because marijuana contains more than 80 known cannabinoids that have been shown to affect different parts of the brain and body, various strains (which contain different concentrations of cannabinoids) can induce different results. In order to plan the best marijuana experience possible, you should understand as much as possible how each strain impacts you personally.

Summary of Effects:

Energy

Generally speaking, sativa strains tend to contain higher levels of THC, or the primary psychoactive component in marijuana. Sativa-dominant strains are much more likely to promote energy and creative thinking. Sativa strains tend to evoke conversation. It is important to note, however, that high doses of many sativas, especially those with THC levels over 18 percent, may promote anxiety or paranoia in some individuals. Most strains have about 15% THC at the upper limits.

Sleep

There are multiple factors that contribute to the soporific, or sleep-inducing, effect of marijuana. One of which is how Indica-dominant the particular strain is. Strains that favor

Indica characteristics will therefore cause a much more predictable sleepy sensation which can be used to treat insomnia and sleep apnea. Another factor to consider when searching for the best strains for sleep is the presence of the cannabinoid, cannabinol (CBN). CBN, known for promoting sleep, is a product of cannabis degeneration and can therefore be created by allowing your favorite strain to dry out a bit in the sun. This will cause the THCa (which is usually converted to THC with heat) to transform into CBNa which will transform into CBN when it becomes heated.

Pain Management

There are many components in marijuana that contribute to its analgesic effects. THC, for example, has been shown to significantly reduce pain in cancer patients by binding with pain-sensing receptors in the body. But it isn't just THC that promotes pain management. Another exciting cannabinoid, CBD, has also been shown to reduce pain and inflammation without causing the characteristic "high" produced by THC. This cannabinoid works in conjunction with THC and other cannabinoids to relieve pain and restore tissue.

Anxiety

Researchers have confirmed that low doses of THC can lower anxiety levels in mice models by binding with CB1 receptors in the amygdala, or the part of the brain responsible for feelings of stress and anxiety. Chronic stress or trauma has been shown to reduce natural endocannabinoid production, which may contribute to prolonged feelings of anxiety. According to one study, THC may reduce anxiety by stimulating CB1 receptors in the amygdala and supplementing phytocannabinoids (cannabinoids derived from plants) for the missing endocannabinoids. Taken in higher doses, however, THC seems to have the opposite effect. Instead of reducing anxiety, high levels of THC might actually make matters worse by reducing the efficiency of cannabinoid receptors. Those who wish to treat (or avoid) anxiety during their marijuana experience should choose strains with low THC levels and higher CBD levels, which has been shown to both reduce anxiety and counter the effects of THC.

Strains are diverse and vast in their cannabinoid content. Here is the top 10 of all Medical Strains list and then will list the approved conditions in Arkansas and the best strains for those conditions based on cannabinoid content.

1. Arvidekal (insomnia): +++CBD (15-20%)/+THC(1%)

2. Afgan Kush (insomnia/anxiety): +++THC (20%)

3. Charlotte's Web (seizures- named after a girl named Charlotte that had severe epilepsy): +++CBD (20%)/+THC (0.5%)

4. Girl Scout Cookies- (pain/migraine): +++THC(20%)

5. One to One (muscle spasms): 1:1 THC/CBD

6. ACDC (alternative cannabinoid dietary cannabis for IBS, inflammation, super food, migraine, fibromyalgia): ++++CBD

7. Strawberry cough (depression): +++THC (20%)

8. Harlequin (pain/mental health/depression): 5:2 THC/CBD

9. Stress Killer (daytime stress): +++CBD/+THC(11%)

10. Zensation (hybrid for pain management and insomnia) ++++THC (24%)

For Arkansas qualifying conditions these are strains that you may inquire at your dispensary about:

- Cancer - https://www.leafly.com/explore/conditions-cancer Harlequin, Purple Kush, God's Gift
- Glaucoma- https://www.leafly.com/explore/conditions-glaucoma Jupiter OG, Santa Maria,Buddha Tahoe
- HIV/AIDS - https://www.leafly.com/explore/conditions-hivaids Blue mystic, Apple Kush, Lemon Bubble
- Hepatitis C - https://www.midwestcompassion.org/2015/05/19/treating-hepatitis-c-with-cannabis/ Northern Lights
- ALS or Lou Gehrig's Disease - https://cannasos.com/strains/conditions/als- cali dream, blue dream, super sour deisel
- Tourette's Syndrome - https://www.leafly.com/explore/conditions-tourettes-syndrome Shiskaberry, Jr, Superman OG
- Crohn's disease/Ulcerative colitis - https://www.leafly.com/explore/conditions-crohns-disease Dr Who, Black Domino, Nebula
- Post-traumatic Stress Disorder (PTSD) - https://www.leafly.com/explore/conditions-ptsd Blue dream, sour diesel, Girl Scout Cookies
- Severe arthritis - https://www.leafly.com/explore/conditions-arthritis Blue Dream, Gorilla Glue#4, BubbaKush
- Fibromyalgia/Chronic pain- https://www.leafly.com/explore/symptoms-pain Blue dream, sour diesel, Girl Scout cookies
- Alzheimer's disease - https://www.leafly.com/explore/symptoms-alzheimers Skunk no.1, Green Monster, Green Haze
- A chronic or debilitating disease that produces:
- Cachexia or wasting syndrome - https://www.leafly.com/explore/symptoms-cachexia Grapefruit haze, El nino, Urkle Train Haze
- Peripheral neuropathy - https://cannabis.net/blog/medical/neuropathy-and-medical-marijuana-strain-guide White widow, Purple Kush, Chemdawg
- Intractable pain - https://www.leafly.com/explore/symptoms-pain Blue dream, sour diesel, Girl Scout Cookies
- Severe nausea - https://www.leafly.com/explore/symptoms-nausea Cheese, God's Gift, Agent Orange
- Seizures, including those characteristic of epilepsy - https://www.leafly.com/explore/symptoms-seizures Grapefruit Kush, Purple Berry, Kushberry
- Severe or persistent muscle spasms, including those characteristic of multiple sclerosis - https://www.leafly.com/explore/symptoms-muscle-spasms Chocolope, Death Star, Platinum Girl Scout Cookies

Chapter 6

Consumable Options

If you are in one of the states where marijuana has recently been legalized, you might believe that your only way to get your medications is to start smoking or using a marijuana vaporizer. You may well be surprised to learn that somewhere between 40 and 50% of all marijuana-based sales in the United States are actually in edible form. This is great news for the people who want to try marijuana, but who have never smoked or used a vape pen. This is actually a problem for people suffering from ailments that they know could be helped with the consumption of marijuana. Here are the common ways to consume Medical Cannabis with the pros and cons.

This easy guide is intended to help patients and caregivers understand the different method of administration of medical marijuana, so that they can make educated decision about the products they purchase and try.

Medical cannabis is a very effective medicine used by patients across the globe to treat and alleviate symptoms of many serious medical conditions that do not respond to traditional interventions. Studies have proven that cannabis has therapeutic properties that cannot be replicated by any other currently prescribed medications, and it induces far fewer and much less severe side effects than many commonly prescribed pharmaceuticals and over the counter drugs.

Smoking Medical Cannabis

How it works: Pack a small amount of dried (cured) cannabis flower into a pipe, water pipe (bong), or rolling paper (to create a "joint"). Then hold a flame to the cannabis flower until it combusts as you inhale the smoke from the mouthpiece or other end of the joint.

Dosage: Start small! Inhale lightly. There is no need to hold the smoke in your lung, exhale, wait a few minutes. If you don't feel the desired effect, or you want to feel a greater effect, take another hit.

Vaporizing ``Vaping`` Medical Marijuana

How it works: Preheat the vaporizer to the recommended temperature. Insert a small amount of dried (cured) cannabis flower or extract into a vaporizer. Press the button and inhale. The cannabis will be heated to a temperature below its combustion point, but still hot enough to release the medicinal compounds. Vaporizers are available in a wide array of shapes and sizes, from fancy home units to pocket-friendly pens.

Medical Marijuana Edibles

How it works: Once upon a time, edibles were limited to homemade brownies that tasted pretty awful and contained a mystery dose of THC. Nowadays you can find medicated cookies, popcorn, crackers, nut mixes, lollipops, ice cream, gummy bears, chocolate bars, chews, and many other kinds of food. The culinary science has evolved enough that most products are delicious and you can hardly tell they contain cannabis.

Dosage: Only use edibles under the supervision of a doctor. Dosages vary widely depending on your weight, metabolism, experience level, and other factors. Doctors we know have suggested starting with a small amount—2 mg or less—and waiting at least an hour before eating more.

Tinctures or Sub-Lingual Sprays

How it works: Extracted cannabinoids are mixed into an alcohol, glycerin solution or MCT Oil (Medium-Chain Triglyceride), which in many cases is coconut oil. These sublingual products usually come in a small bottle. Just squirt or spray it under your tongue and let it absorb through the thin tissue of the mouth.

Dosage: Start with just a few drops and wait ten minutes. If you don't feel relief, try a few more drops. Eventually you'll figure out your ideal dosage for most people, it's between half a dropper and a couple of droppers at a time.

Transdermal Patches

How it works: Apply patch to a clean, dry and hairless skin surface. Many medical professionals recommend adhering the patch on the inner-wrist area, top of foot or ankle. This is the ideal method for any patients who rather not inhale the medicine. If you have explored multiple options without success, this might be the right path for depending on your choice of high you are trying to reach.

Dosage: Most transdermal patches come in 10mg dosed patches. They can be cut in half for smaller doses.

<u>Suppositories</u>

How it works: You insert a small cone-shaped mass of cannabis extract into the rectum, where it absorbs through the colon. This method is somewhat controversial and rather less dignified than other ways to medicate, but some patients swear by it. Put on protective gloves, lie on your side, and insert the suppository about 1.5 inches. Squeeze your sphincter muscles and stay in place for at least a few minutes. When you're ready, get up, throw away the gloves, and thoroughly wash your hands. There are also companies who make pre-made ratios of medicine for rectal use – 1 mg non-injectable syringes.

Dosage: Most suppositories come in two sizes: 2g for adults and 1g for children. They can be cut in half for smaller doses.

<u>Topicals</u>

How it works: Medical cannabis tinctures are a great way to medicate without any psychoactive effects. Salves, ointments, lotions, and sprays are great for arthritis, chapped skin, eczema, minor burns, muscle soreness, sunburns, swellings, joint pain, and tendonitis, to name just a few.

Dosage: You're unlikely to cause any real harm with topicals, but do try to find ones that are aimed at your specific ailment. Use salves and ointments as much as you want as often as you want, keeping in mind that they can get greasy. If you experience skin irritation, discontinue use. Consult your doctor about using transdermal patches.

<u>Ingesting Fresh Medical Cannabis</u>

How it works: Raw cannabis has developed quite a following.

Patients claim that the raw plant has medicinal properties that are lost when the plant is dried or heated. You ingest the raw leaves and buds straight from the plant, usually by mixing them into a juice or smoothie.

Dosage: Dr. William Courtney, the leading advocate of juicing, recommends ingesting fifteen leaves and one or two big buds (2–4″) daily.

Beverages

How it works: Your local dispensary probably sells bottles of cannabis-infused teas, juices, smoothies, and sodas. You can also make your own cannabis tea by steeping a bud, piece of wax, or tincture in hot water. Adding a bag of your favorite tea can improve its flavor. Hemp (Cannabis) leaf in cup of tea.

Dosage: Consult with your doctor before drinking marijuana beverages. Start with one small sip & wait an hour before deciding whether or not to drink more.

Dabbing

How it works: A "dab" is a cannabis concentrate (hash oil, budder, shatter, wax, etc.) that you heat to a high temperature and inhale. The delivery devices vary, but they tend to be complicated and usually involve the use of a butane torch. Also, concentrates can contain as much as 90 percent THC, so you will get a very high dose of psychoactive compounds. This method is NOT recommended for patients with a low THC tolerance or those new to cannabis medications!

Dosage: Consult with your doctor prior to trying dabbing, it's probably more than you need. If you do choose to try it, start with just one 'small' hit, but know that it will have extremely strong psychoactive effects.

	Pros	Cons
Smoking	<ul><li>Delivers instant relief</li><li>Fairly easy to regulate dosage</li><li>Inexpensive</li><li>Minimally processed</li><li>Multiple options</li></ul>	<ul><li>Smoke may be harmful to lungs. Studies have reached contradictory, bu combustion of an substance makes harder to breathe</li><li>In many cases, n a good option for anyone with pulmonary dama; (lung cancer, emphysema) or asthma</li><li>Will make you smell like cannab smoke</li></ul>
Vaping	<ul><li>Delivers instant relief</li><li>Less harsh on lungs than smoking</li><li>Doesn't make you smell as much as smoking</li></ul>	<ul><li>Vaping units can be very expensive</li><li>Battery powered units must be recharged.</li><li>Need time to war up device.</li></ul>
Edibles	<ul><li>Provides long-lasting relief.</li><li>Good alternative for people averse to inhaling.</li><li>You get to eat a delicious treat.</li><li>Dosage can be very precise</li></ul>	<ul><li>Can take half an hour to several hours to kick in.</li><li>Dosage can be difficult if the manufacturer.</li><li>Must be locked u to avoid children and pets.</li><li>Causes a differen</li></ul>

	Pros	Cons
		"high" than smoking.
...ctures/Sp...s	• Doesn't hurt lungs like inhaling cannabis. • Easy to control dosage for a very low dose. • Mild taste. • Preferred method for children.	• Can be expensive for people who require a high dosage of cannabinoids. • Takes effect faster than edibles, but still not as fast as inhalation.
...ches	• No Smoking Required. • Comes in different formulations. • Mild dosages.	• Some individuals may develop an allergic reaction. • Must be applied on a clean and dry skin surface. • Not be applied where a great deal of body hair
...ctal ...ppository	• Great alternative to edibles. • Kicks in quickly and lasts long • Most Efficient way to digest.	• Difficult and embarrassing to administer. • Must be refrigerated. • Difficult to apply.
...picals	• Topicals don't get you "high" • Addresses skin issues • Localized pain relief	• Does not help cancer, PTSD, epilepsy, or glaucoma. • Don't provide a euphoric feeling. • Patients report some products simply don't work.
...gesting ...w	• Raw cannabis is packed with THC-A, the acid form of THC, which is not psychoactive. Some patients and doctors believe THC-A has unique medicinal	• Requires large amounts of fresh cannabis. • May have an unpleasant

	properties. • Some patients whose chronic diseases never responded to other treatment (including dried cannabis) say that juicing raw marijuana has been their miracle cure.	vegetable taste. • Studies have no confirmed resul
Beverages	• Provides long-lasting relief. • Alternative for people averse to inhaling their medicine. • Give a specific feeling, such as stress relief or energy.	• Takes 30min-2hours to kick i • Dosage can be difficult. • Causes a differe "high" than smoking.
Dabbing	• Useful for urgent medication of acute illnesses. • Cost-efficient for patients who need High-THC. • Provides instant relief.	• Concentrates ar higher risk of containing harn chemicals. • Solvents are use to extract the medicinal chemicals, may not be properly removed. • May cause overdose, while never fatal, can very unpleasant and uncomfortable.

Chapter 8

How To Obtain Legally in Your State (Arkansas)

As of 2017 and the writing of this book, patients can now apply for medical marijuana identification cards in the state of Arkansas. However, possession and use of recreational marijuana is still illegal. Medical marijuana doctors in Arkansas provide recommendations for patients deemed eligible for medical cannabis, who then visit dispensaries to obtain medical marijuana. Most Arkansas dispensaries provide different cannabis strains for medicinal use, such as Sativa, hybrids and Indica.

Under Arkansas statutes, people with valid recommendations from their Arkansas medical marijuana doctor can possess no more than 2.5 ounces of cannabis at one time. In addition, medical marijuana patients must qualify for an Arkansas MMJ card before they can purchase medical cannabis at a dispensary.

The Arkansas Department of Finance and Administration is expected to issue additional guidelines regarding the recent passing of the Medical Marijuana Amendment. These guidelines should include rules about the sale and cultivation of medical cannabis as well as additional information specifically for Arkansas marijuana doctors.

According to Issue 6, medical conditions qualifying for recommendations from medical marijuana doctors in Arkansas include:

- Posttraumatic stress disorder
- Cancer
- Tourette's syndrome
- ALS (Lou Gehrig's disease)
- Glaucoma
- Ulcerative colitis
- Hepatitis C
- HIV/AIDS
- Severe arthritis
- Crohn's disease
- Fibromyalgia
- Alzheimer's disease
- Wasting syndrome (cachexia)
- Seizures
- Debilitating/chronic diseases

Medical marijuana patients in Arkansas will not be able to grow cannabis at home. Arkansas medical cannabis dispensaries will be permitted to deliver MMJ to patients with recommendations from their Arkansas marijuana doctor. In addition, Arkansas plans to tax medical marijuana sales in accordance with local and state sales tax laws.

When Arkansas begins initiating their medical marijuana program, MarijuanaDoctors.com will have a list of all verified MMJ doctors as well as legally operating dispensaries. MMJ users can then check out each listing to view location, business hours, delivery information, customer satisfaction reviews and other details pertinent to receiving the best medical cannabis available in Arkansas.

The Arkansas Department of Health issues medical marijuana registry cards for qualified patients and caregivers.

Information and forms are required when a patient applies for a Medical Marijuana ID card:

- The completed Physician Written Certification

- Photocopy of your Arkansas issued driver's license or state ID (remember: name and address must match what is listed on your Arkansas driver's license or ID)

- The nonrefundable $50 application fee.

In November 2016 Arkansas voters approved medical marijuana through the passage of a constitutional amendment, known as Amendment 98, the Arkansas Medical Marijuana Act of 2016. The law allows qualifying patients to purchase and use medical marijuana from a licensed dispensary if certain criteria are met. One of the requirements is a physician certification of qualifying conditions.

Physicians are not required to complete and sign the certification for a patient; only physicians who choose to participate.

If a physician is willing to complete a physician certification form for a patient to use medical marijuana obtained from a licensed dispensary, a physician must sign the form.

Your physician will certifying that they have completed an in-person patient assessment.

That the patient DOES have one of the qualifying conditions.

That they are licensed to practice in Arkansas.

That they have a current DEA number.

That they currently do not accept federal health insurance

There is an approved form from the Arkansas Department of Health (ADH).

This form cannot be substituted with a letter or other type of certification.

This form is available to print from the ADH website. You can make blank copies of the form.

Any medical doctor or doctor of osteopathy licensed to practice in Arkansas with a current DEA number is authorized to sign the form.

There is no specific medical marijuana training required by law in order to complete the form.

Completing the form:

All portions of the form must be filled out completely.

Do not leave the form blank anywhere in the content areas.

Complete the patient demographic portion at the top of the form. Patient must be an Arkansas resident.

Identify if the patient is disabled or under the age of 18.

This is necessary for determining their need for a certified caregiver who will be authorized by law to purchase and transport medical marijuana for the patient.

Check the correct time frame box for the patient. It may be up to 12 months, or less depending on your determination for the patient.

Fully fill out all physician information. Do not leave any portion blank.

The patient or patient's guardian must also sign the form.

The form has a complete list of the qualifying conditions.

No other conditions are approved at this time.(New conditions are added by rule change of the Arkansas Board of Health).

ADH will not accept applications that have additional write-in conditions.

The agency may contact the physician to verify the signature.

Physician's license & DEA number will be verified.

You should keep a record of the visit.

The physician certification form may be copied and placed in the patient's medical record as part of your documentation.

All aspects of this process are covered by HIPAA.

You may complete a certification for a minor who has a qualifying condition.

The parent/guardian must be present and they must sign the form.

Remember to certify that the patient is under 18 on the form.

A designated caregiver is a person who may purchase and transport medical marijuana from an Arkansas dispensary, for a qualified patient who is either a minor or is physically disabled.

Minors are required to have a parent/ guardian as a designated caregiver. Physically disabled patients may have one if they so choose.

Designations of age or physical disability must be marked on the certification form.

Physicians do not have to see a caregiver unless the patient is a minor, and then they must review the form with the minor patient's parent/guardian.

The applicant will send the certification to ADH as part of their application. They may do this via mail, or through ADH's online application system.

The physician certification is valid for 30 days.

If a patient gets a certification and fails to submit it to ADH within 30 days, they must get a new certification.

A patient's registration identification card is valid for one year from issuance.

If you as the physician wish for the patient's registration identification card to be valid for less than one year, please note that on the form in the area marked "issue registry card for."

The patient must submit their completed application online or via mail.

The application is reviewed and it is either approved or denied.

If all requirements are met, a registry card will be issued.

The card will expire based on the date recommended on the physician certification.

How to Request and Obtain Your Medical Records

Before your marijuana evaluation appointment, it's imperative that you obtain a copy of your medical records, indicating your diagnosis. In order to get medical marijuana in any state, you must first obtain a copy of your medical records.

If you arrive to your appointment without these records, your marijuana doctor will likely be able to request the records on your behalf, but this will delay the process of obtaining the medical marijuana recommendation needed to use cannabis legally in your state. It's quick and easy to obtain your medical records, and it will help you get medical marijuana sooner.

Step 1: Contact Your Primary Care Doctor

Most practices require you to fill out a specific form to formally request your medical records. To obtain this form, simply call your primary care doctor's office, or the office of the doctor who gave you the diagnosis, and request a copy. They should be able to deliver it to you by fax, email, postal mail or you may pick it up from the doctor's office.

If the doctor's office doesn't have a specific form, simply write a letter to request your records. Be sure to include:

Your name, including your maiden name (if applicable)

Social security number

Date of birth

Address and phone number

Email address

Record(s) being requested

Dates you were under the doctor's care

Signature

Delivery option (pick up, fax, email, etc.)

What if I Don't Have a Primary Care Doctor?

If you do not have a primary care doctor, are uninsured, have not had a check-up in a while, or cannot afford to see a physician, your medical marijuana doctor may be able to assist in finding an affordable clinic in your area that can give you an exam and diagnosis. Or, in some cases, your marijuana doctor may be able to take you on as a new patient and provide a diagnosis for you. In California and Colorado, patients may be issued a temporary recommendation pending the acquisition of medical records.

Step 2: Bring Medical Records to Your Marijuana Evaluation Appointment

Remember to bring your medical records form to your medical marijuana evaluation appointment. These documents are imperative to continuing your care with MarijuanaDoctors.com and receiving a medical marijuana recommendation in every state.

You can apply online by going to
http://www.healthy.arkansas.gov/programs-services/topics/medical-marijuana

Patient Seeking Medical Cannabis ID Card PROCESS

Online application: Home | Apply Online | FAQs | Forms | Patient Info | Caregiver Info

In order to qualify for a registry card to legally purchase medical marijuana, you must meet the following qualifications:

- Be 18 years of age or older or be a minor patient with parental consent.

- Be diagnosed with a qualifying medical condition – SEE LIST

- and any other medical condition or its treatment approved by the Department of Health

- Have the official written certification from a physician.

- Be an Arkansas resident with proof of residency. (AR Driver's License or AR State ID card).

- State law prohibits members of Arkansas National Guard and United States Military from obtaining a registry ID card.

Steps to Get Started and Items Needed

Step 1 – Physician Written Certification Form

Arkansas Department of Health
Medical Marijuana Physician Written Certification

Patient Information

First Name	MI	Last Name	

Street Number and Street Name (or PO Box)

Unit Number	Unit Type (Apt, Unit, Suite, etc.)

City	State	Zip Code

Date of Birth (MM/DD/YYYY)	Under the age of 18?	Physically Disabled?
	◯ Yes ◯ No	◯ Yes ◯ No

X
___ I hold a valid, unrestricted, existing license to practice as a medical physician or osteopathic physician in
X Arkansas.
___ It is my professional opinion, after having completed an in-person assessment of the patient's medical
history and current medical condition in the course of a physician patient relationship, the patient has a
qualifying medical condition identified below.

Select the qualifying medical condition(s):

- ☐ Cancer
- ☐ Glaucoma
- ☐ Positive status for human immunodeficiency virus/ acquired immune deficiency syndrome
- ☐ Hepatitis C
- ☐ Amyotrophic lateral sclerosis
- ☐ Tourette's syndrome
- ☐ Crohn's disease
- ☐ Ulcerative colitis
- ☐ Post-traumatic stress disorder
- ☐ Severe arthritis
- ☐ Fibromyalgia
- ☐ Alzheimer's disease
- ☐ Cachexia or wasting syndrome
- ☐ Peripheral neuropathy
- ☐ Intractable pain, which is pain that has not responded to ordinary medications, treatment or surgical measures for more than six (6) months
- ☐ Severe nausea
- ☐ Seizures, including without limitation those characteristic of epilepsy
- ☐ Severe and persistent muscle spasms, including without limitation those characteristic of multiple sclerosis

Issue Registry Card for: ◉ 12 Months   ◯ Less than 12 months ___ Months ___ Weeks

Physician Information

First Name	MI	Last Name	Suffix
Tammy	J	Tucker	D.O.

Arkansas Medical License Number	DEA Number
E3741	BT7582972

Address
6203 WILLOW CREEK DR

Unit Number	Unit Type (Apt, Unit, Suite, etc.)
	Suite 2

City	State	Zip Code
Springdale	AR	72762

Phone	I do hereby attest that this information is true, accurate and complete.	Signature	Date
1-800-479-6435			

The information in this certification is correct as to the patient or parent, custodian, legal guardian, by signing I indicate I am aware of this diagnosis and medical marijuana physician written certification and authorize the Arkansas Department of Health to verify as warranted.

◉ Patient ◯ Parent ◯ Custodian ◯ Legal Guardian   Signature   Date

Print Name

The first step to getting a medical marijuana registry card in Arkansas is to meet with your physician about medical marijuana. Your physician must be licensed to practice in Arkansas and have a current DEA number. If your physician agrees to complete the Physician Certification Form, you will upload it with your patient application or mail it with your application depending on which method you choose. The Physician Written Certification expires 30 days from the date it was signed by the physician. You must upload or mail the form with your application before it expires. If you allow a physician certification form to expire, the certification becomes invalid and you will no longer be able to use it with your registry application.

Step 2 – Fill Out the Patient Application

Arkansas Department of Health
Medical Marijuana Registry Patient Application

Patient Information | ☐ **New Application** | ☐ **Renewal**

First Name | MI | Last Name | Phone

Mailing Address

Street Number and Street Name (or PO Box)

Unit Number | Unit Type (Apt, Unit, Suite, etc.)

City | State | Zip Code

Residence Address (If different from mailing address) | ☐ **Check if homeless**

Street Number and Street Name

Unit Number | Unit Type (Apt, Unit, Suite etc.)

City | State | Zip

Date of Birth (MM/DD/YYYY) | Sex ☐ Male ☐ Female | Race | Eye Color | Height | Physically Disabled ☐ Yes ☐ No

Arkansas DL or ID Number | Expiration Date (MM/DD/YYYY) | Last 4 digits of SSN | Registry ID (for renewals only)

☐ Yes ☐ No   Are you a member of the Arkansas National Guard or the United States military?

By signing, I, the patient pledge not to divert marijuana to anyone who is not allowed to possess marijuana under the Arkansas Medical Marijuana Amendment of 2016

Signature | Date

Print Name

Parent / Guardian / Legal Custodian -- Skip if applicant over 18

First Name | MI | Last Name | Phone

Address

Unit Number | Unit Type (Apt, Unit, Suite, etc.)

City | State | Zip Code

By signing, I confirm that I, as the parent/guardian/legal custodian allow the qualifying patient's medical use of marijuana, will assist the qualifying patient in the medical use of marijuana and will control the acquisition of the marijuana, dosage and the frequency of the medical use of marijuana by the qualifying patient and will register as a designated caregiver.

Signature | ☐ Parent ☐ Custodian ☐ Legal Guardian | Date

Print Name

20170727

Complete the patient application in its entirety. Name and address must match what is listed on the state ID provided.

If you will require a caregiver, ensure that the caregiver completes a caregiver application.

Step 3 – Pay the Application Fee (nonrefundable)

The fee is $50 and is non-refundable for all who apply. If you apply online, there will be a section for payment options. If you are mailing your application, please include a check or money order for $50, payable to the Arkansas Department of Health.

Note: Cash payments will not be accepted.

Step 4 – Submit Proof of Age and Identity

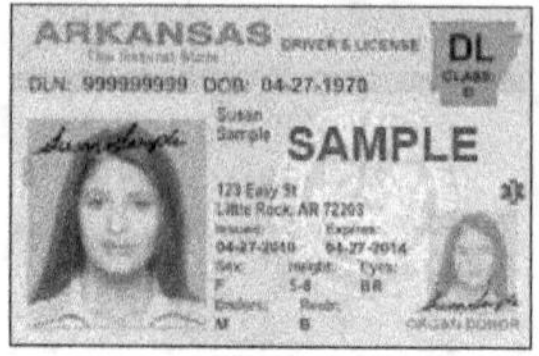

You must upload a copy of your Arkansas issued driver's license or ID with your application. If you're mailing your application, send in a photocopy of your Arkansas issued driver's license or state ID with your application.

Step 5 – Submit Physician's Written Certification

You must upload a copy of your Physician's Written Certification form with your application. If you're mailing your application, send in a photocopy of your Physician's Written Certification form with your application.

If you are mailing your application, send to:

Arkansas Department of Health

Medical Marijuana Section

4815 West Markham Slot 50

Little Rock, AR 72205

Chapter 9

Cannabis and Workplace Rules

The Arkansas Medical Cannabis Act is the newly passed medical marijuana law in Arkansas, which was approved by voters in the 2016 election.

This new law allows individuals with "qualifying medical conditions" to use medical marijuana to treat those conditions.

The new law went into effect on November 9, 2016

The impact on employers?

With this new law, Arkansas created a new protected class around medical marijuana use. Under the new law, employers are prohibited from terminating an employee based on his/her medical marijuana use. In other words, an employer cannot fire an employee simply because he/she has a prescription to use medical marijuana. An employer can, however, terminate an employee for coming to work "high." In addition, the new law does not require employers to accommodate an employee's request to use medical marijuana in the workplace. One thing the law does not address, however, is the use of drug testing (pre-employment, safety-sensitive, or reasonable suspicion) on an employee who uses medical marijuana. Current drug tests only flag whether THC (the active ingredient in marijuana) is present in the individual's system and does not determine the level of a tested individual's impairment. This means that an individual can test positive for marijuana without being "high." It is recommended that employers train frontline supervisors and managers will need to be more vigilant about documenting independent indications of impairment in the workplace such as unusual sleepiness, slowed perception and motor skills, and red eyes.

Arkansas does have a "Drug Free Workplace Program" through the State Labor Department which gives incentives and discounts on worker's comp insurance premiums. The program does discuss drug testing and you can go to http://www.arkansas.gov/government/agency-detail/labor-arkansas-department to learn more.

Chapter 10

Conclusion

Different people have different experiences. One individual may feel stress release, while another feels over-stimulated and stressed, while another feels energized and on-task. There are many factors that impact the effect:

- Amount used (dosage)
- Strain of cannabis used and method of consumption
- Environment/setting
- Experience and history of cannabis use
- Biochemistry
- Mindset or mood
- Nutrition or diet
- Types of Cannabis

All types of medical cannabis produce effects that are more similar than not, including pain and nausea control, appetite stimulation, reduced muscle spasm, improved sleep, and others. But individual strains will have differing cannabinoid and terpene content, producing noticeably different effects. Many people report finding some strains more beneficial than others. For instance, strains with more CBD tend to produce better pain and spasticity relief. As noted above, effects will also vary for an individual based on the setting in which it is used and the person's physiological state when using it.

Knowledge is Power!

Appendix

Suggested Websites for More Information

https://www.leafly.com/

https://unitedpatientsgroup.com

http://herb.co/

https://www.coloradopotguide.com/

https://www.marijuanadoctors.com/

http://www.safeaccessnow.org/using_medical_cannabis

Patient Stories and Testimonials

My name is Elise Lewis I have A.D.D. and generalized anxiety disorder. I was raised in a home where we didn't take medicine; the only thing we took was a Tylenol if we had a fever. So I was never put on any medication for my A.D.D. or anxiety. Which was fine really, although, I have struggled with these I have found ways to cope and maintain a normal life. Even though I am 95% against all medications I am pro marijuana. I do not smoke marijuana or do any other drugs I don't even drink alcohol but I back marijuana 100%.

Let's talk about CBD, we have all heard stories and seen videos of CBD helping with seizures, Alzheimer's, anxiety, pain management, the list goes on and on. I had no idea though that I was able to get CBD through the mail and at some local distributors, I thought you had to have a medical card and live in a state that allowed medical marijuana. I decided it was time I tried some of this stuff. I was curious to see how it would help my anxiety. I didn't dream it would do all it has done for me.

I own a cleaning business. I have 4 employees and we have many cleaning accounts. It is hard enough for a normal person to deal with the stresses of owning a business but for a girl with A.D.D. and severe anxiety, it's unbearable at times.

Anxiety is always there, I am always very tense. So, on a day to day basis I have many anxiety attacks, I panic when driving, I panic when something is taking too long, such as waiting in line or I concentrate to long on what I am doing. I get anxiety in groups of people, I avoid crowds and restaurants at all costs. I only get food through the drive thru, never go in to sit down. I have missed out on my son's field trips, enjoying nice dinners out, I've had to leave in the middle of movies at the theater, parties, family get togethers, anxiety was getting in the way of life. I am also a nail biter. It is the worst when watching tv or a movie and when driving. The second I sit down my fingers are in my mouth. My husband had to constantly tell me to stop. It was a habit (or so I thought) something I did without realizing it.

The mind of a person with A.D.D. is very complicated haha. I am one of the most forgetful people you will ever know. I have always thought I have short term memory loss. I have to have routines if I am thrown off my routine it throws me completely off and my entire day will be off. I have to constantly run my schedule for the day through my head. Literally all day I am saying, "Farm 8-10, 15 mins home, eat breakfast , get stuff together, leave at 9:45, get to next job at 10:30…." And so on and so forth. Literally I repeat the schedule to myself all day every day so I won't forget. I don't read and comprehend; I have 1,000's of things running through my head at once. I cannot concentrate on a sentence and know what it says. I have to read it multiple times, often times I have to take a nap after reading a few paragraphs because the intense concentration I have to use to comprehend the words exhausts me.

Then there is the back pain, which I had no idea the CBD would help with it. The pain is so intense that I thought my bones were deformed and surgery was my only option. We had to turn our mattress every other night, truly every 2 days, because I would wake up with such severe pain. Turns out it wasn't the mattress.

Now that you know a bit about me and how I've functioned day to day my whole life, let's talk about how I now function while taking CBD. On the first day I took the CBD I felt very relaxed. I felt the pressure of work and life just melt away. I found myself not rushing everywhere, I didn't feel like I had do every task on my list all at the same time. The day slowed down. There is no THC in CBD oil so there is no high, just throwing that out there HAHA. I get all of my work done during the day surprisingly faster than before because I am not stressing over every little thing. That first week I had spent almost 200 dollars eating out because I was actually going into restaurants and sitting down and eating. This is unheard of ya'll. I did not care at all that it was lunch hour I wanted to be in a restaurant. The anxiety was completely gone. I had only one brief feeling of anxiety in the past month.

As far as my A.D.D. symptoms go. I have none, my memory has drastically improved and my mind has slowed down. I can think, I can read and comprehend, I can carry on conversations and actually hear and understand and respond. It is absolutely amazing.

I was sitting with my husband watching a movie and he asked me, " Are you consciously keeping yourself from biting your nails?" I told him, "no I just don't feeling like biting." I have finger nails now you guys. I haven't chewed on my nails from the very first day of taking CBD.

Lastly, I didn't realize it was helping my back pain, it had been probably 3 weeks when my husband brought it to my attention that we had been sleeping in the same spot for over 3 weeks and I had not one time had any back pain. That in its self is a miracle.

ABOUT THE AUTHOR

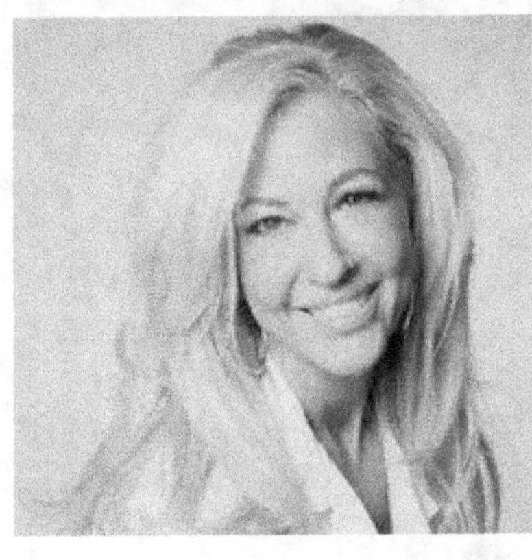

Dr. Tammy Post

Wellness and functional medicine doctor, Hormone Expert (lovingly known as the "Hormone Queen"), author and Spokesperson Dr. Tammy Post (referred to as Dr. Tammy) is a board-certified family physician and founder of multiple programs of health, wellness and lifestyle. As a speaker, Dr. Tammy empowers and inspires those who attend her speaking engagements to do something different to achieve the healthy lifestyle they desire. www.betterlivingrx.com